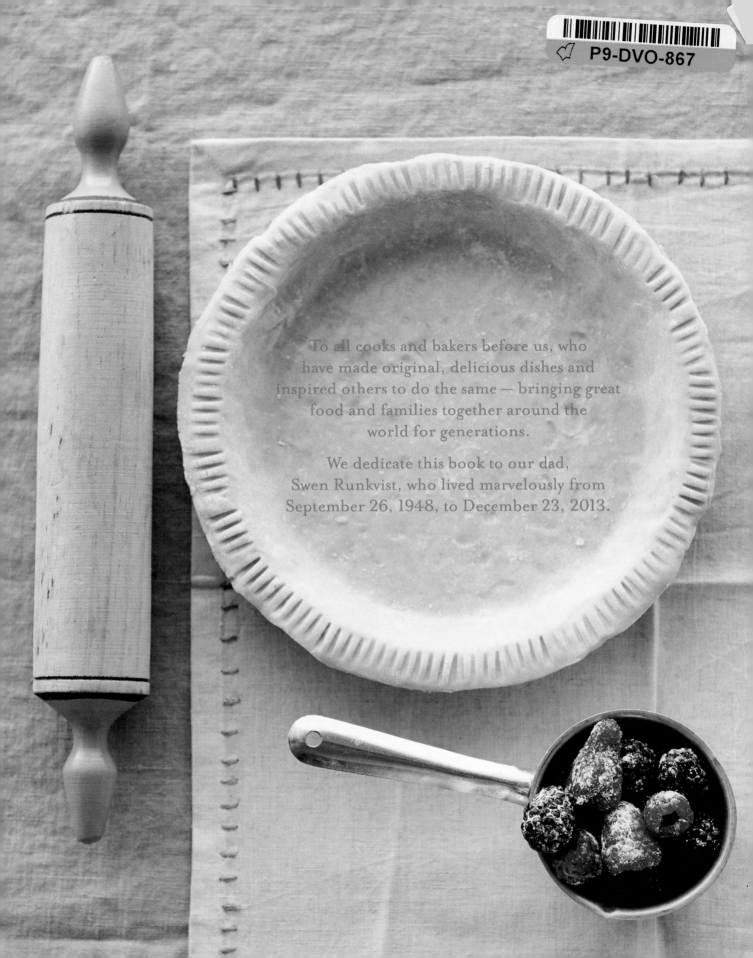

To all cooks and bakers before us, who have made original, delicious dishes and inspired others to do the same — bringing great food and families together around the world for generations.

We dedicate this book to our dad, Swen Runkvist, who lived marvelously from September 26, 1948, to December 23, 2013.

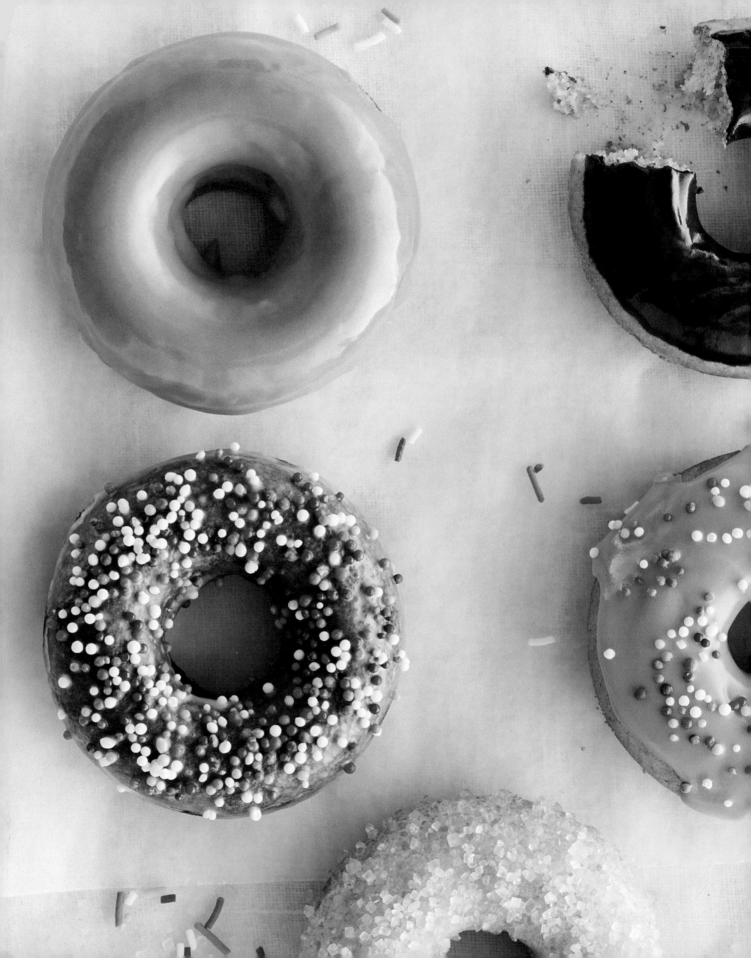

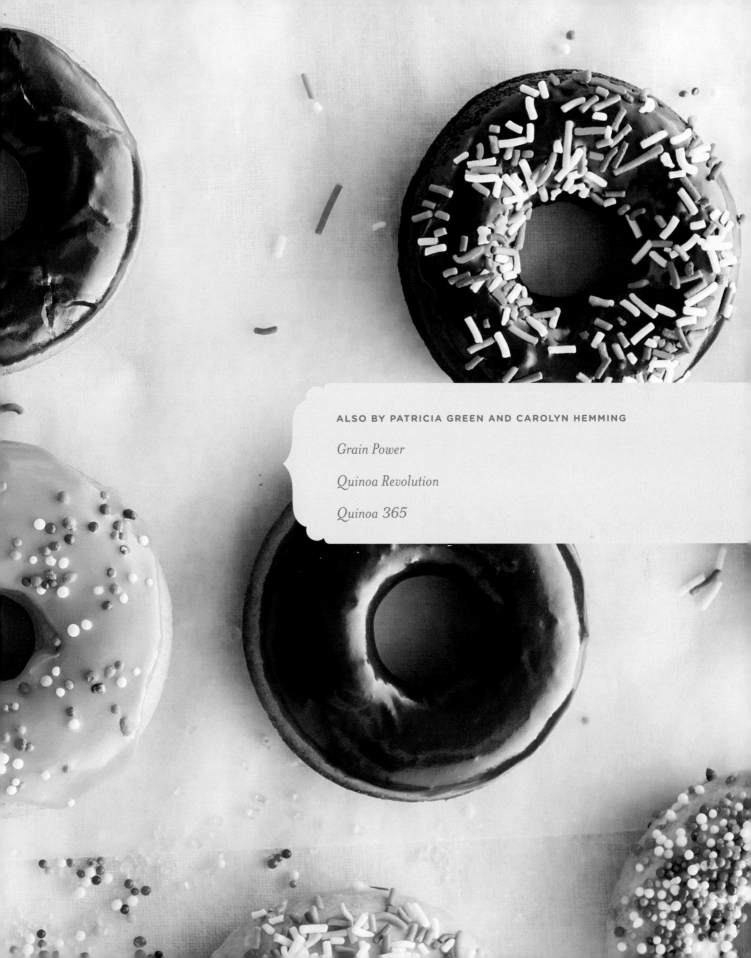

ALSO BY PATRICIA GREEN AND CAROLYN HEMMING

Grain Power

Quinoa Revolution

Quinoa 365

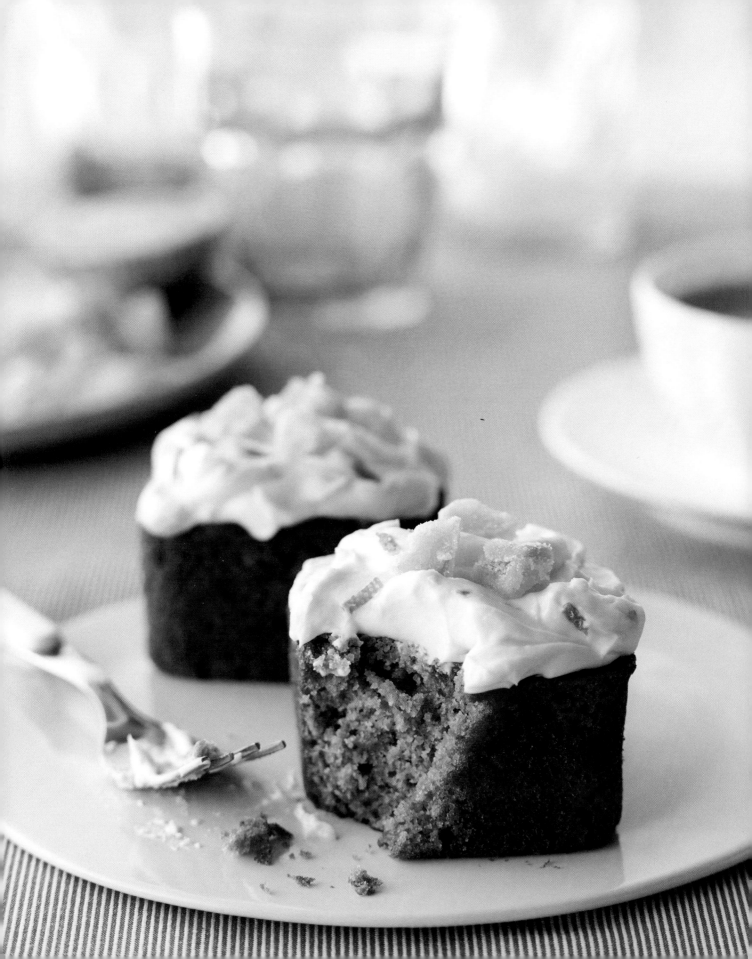

Contents

Introduction   x

Essentials of Gluten-Free Baking   xviii

Cookies, Bars and Squares   1

Cakes, Loaves, Muffins and More   43

Tarts and Pies   99

Special Occasion Baking   129

Savory Breads and Buns   159

Acknowledgments   185

Popular Gluten-Free Ingredients   188

References   195

Index   196

Happy Baking!

Introduction

In the loud grade-school lunchroom that smelled of pudding cups and processed cheese, we felt like outcasts with our homemade, rough-cut sandwich slabs of bread filled with grains and seeds. Over the years, our whining ceased as we recognized that Mom was treating us to something special that most kids never had. For us, homemade cookies, breads, buns, cakes and pastries were the norm, and something our mom prided herself on. There was nothing good about those "factory cookies," she would remind us. The reason she spent any spare evening hours after work kneading, punching and rising dough, scooping cookies or rolling pastry was simple to her: less processed meant more nutritious. Made yourself with whole foods meant you knew exactly what was inside. And she was right.

While we may not always grind our own flour or have farmers down the road who sell eggs, we do have access to quality ingredients and still bake these childhood treats ourselves. With an increasing selection of ingredients available today (including organic) we can expand our creativity to still maintain some nutrition and enjoy that fresh, home-baked treat. We have included a mix of healthier everyday treats as well as some special baking that is richer and intended for special occasions. When you grab a baked snack, wouldn't you like to know what's inside and that there may even be something good in it, even if it's just a rare treat? With these easy recipes we hope you will enjoy the wonderful taste and goodness of home-baking with ancient grains. And don't forget Mom's principle: food is medicine and meant to be taken in moderation (especially treats).

Baking homemade gluten-free treats can be easy! Which is lucky, because store-bought gluten-free baked products may not always be what they're cracked up to be. Today's mass production of consumer foods and ingredients, including those that are gluten-free, means they are usually over-processed and have very little nutrition to offer. Commercially made gluten-free products can be packed with sugar and made almost or completely from starches. The same can be said for many premixed flour blends on the market. There are great benefits to baking from scratch, using naturally gluten-free, ancient grain superfoods

that are not genetically modified. Adding naturally gluten-free ingredients —
such as dried fruit like cranberries and raisins — as well as nuts and coconut
help to make your recipes tasty and add variety. Cookies, cakes, pastries and
breads can leave out the gluten, offer nutrition — and still provide the same
familiar, tasty baking flavors and textures you expect. After all, if you're
going to eat baking, it should be worth it! A wider range of gluten-free
products and ingredients in the market also means more possibilities for
flavors and texture, so many are enjoying gluten-free simply because of the
increased options for variety and taste.

Who is eating gluten-free? People who want to improve their overall
health are eating gluten-free, as are athletes (both elite and recreational)
and people affected by food allergies, diseases and conditions that impose
strict dietary requirements, including celiac disease, wheat allergies, gluten
sensitivity, autism, ADHD, IBS and Asperger syndrome.

Many of us find we are now cooking for family members, friends and
dinner guests with a myriad of dietary restrictions, food preferences and
eating habits (often based on health-conscious or socially ethical reasons).
Whether you're eating gluten-free because of allergy, disease or illness, or
conscious choice, you need not worry about missing out! We are sure you
can eat just as well as, if not better than, people who aren't eating gluten-
free. There are many alternatives to ingredients that contain gluten, as well
as gluten-free store-bought, processed crackers, cookies, pastries, cakes and
breads. But there is no substitute for homemade baking, and store-bought,
gluten-free processed foods do not come close in taste or nutrition to what
you can make yourself with natural, whole, gluten-free ingredients.

Clever food industry marketing and dieting fads once claimed that
bread, baking and carbohydrate-based foods were bad for us, but this is not
necessarily accurate. We need to remind ourselves that the human brain
needs carbohydrates and most certainly cannot function without
them. At one time our ancestors likely ate baking — including
cookies, cakes and breads — that was full of nutrition.
How is this possible? It contained whole grain,
unmodified, unprocessed goodness, including many
of the ancient grains we haven't been accustomed to
eating but are now coming back into our kitchens.

Rich in vitamins B, K and A and in the minerals iron, calcium, magnesium, phosphorus, potassium, manganese, zinc, selenium and copper, as well as omega-3 and omega-6 fatty acids, gluten-free ancient grains can provide a range of beneficial elements, some you may never have even heard of. Complete proteins, complex carbohydrates, good fats, enzymes, plant sterols, flavonoids (phytonutrients), antioxidants, dietary fiber, prebiotics, beta glucans, policosanols and resistant starches are some of the goodies on offer.

Gluten-free ancient grains can help to lower cholesterol and blood pressure, inhibit inflammation, prevent heart disease and stroke, suppress appetite, prevent cancers, promote alkalinity, stabilize blood sugar, manage diabetes or even help prevent type 2 diabetes, improve immune function, hydrate intestines and promote good digestion and nutrient absorption, metabolize fats, repair body tissues, prevent childhood asthma, increase serotonin, prevent upper respiratory symptoms, promote quick healing, prevent bone and muscle loss, prevent gallstones, soothe skin conditions and prevent tumor growth and macular degeneration — to name just a few of their helpful properties. Many whole foods not only are naturally gluten-free with tremendous nutritive value to offer, but also have characteristics that make them ideal ingredients in cooking and baking today. So why not use them?

Whether you must be or are choosing to be gluten-free, processed, packaged, gluten-free foods are not the solution and may not be the best for your health. Simply being labeled "gluten-free" does not make processed and packaged foods automatically healthy. Over-processed ingredients and fillers can lack important vitamins, minerals and fiber and offer no real nutritional value. Some processed, gluten-free ingredients may even have negative aspects such as being high in calories, sugar, salt, fat and additives that can cause poor digestion leading to constipation, weight gain or even more serious problems. Homemade gluten-free baking is the answer to these processed, poorly nutritive substitutes. All the recipes in this book are made gluten-free, using flours and ingredients that do not contain gluten; however, you need to ensure that you purchase ingredients that are processed in gluten-free facilities and are clearly labeled as such on the package. Even foods that are not usually known to contain gluten may have trace amounts or be contaminated by gluten from processing or where they're grown, from proximity or just via circumstances that occur in nature. (For example, oats are often contaminated by gluten, so be aware of this and purchase only products labeled gluten-free.) Also, some ingredients may have come into contact with or contain gluten even though they should not. They may include but are not limited to oats and oat bran, sour cream, baking powder, cornstarch, spices and seasonings, nuts, puffed rice or corn, vanilla extract, powdered (icing) sugar, mayonnaise, chocolates, grated cheese, yogurts, soy products, starches and yeast. Gluten may be indicated on nutritional labels as malt, couscous, farina, bulgur or seitan, or even appear in Latin as hordeum vulgare, triticum vulgare, or secale cereale. Read the labels and be sure.

In the past, inadequate labeling has sometimes caused people to believe that a product actually contains gluten when in fact it has just been contaminated with a source of gluten. Regardless, it all has the same effect, so always make sure that the ingredients you use are consistently labeled as gluten-free and are produced in gluten-free facilities. No matter where you are in the world, whether you're buying by mail order or in your local stores, you should be able to find a wide selection of ingredients that meet gluten-free standards.

Baking can be so satisfying and comforting. Baking at home takes us back to our roots and reminds us of family. The smell of the house when you're baking chocolate chip cookies on a rainy day, baking pies in the fall, baking desserts for all sorts of special occasions or gatherings … It's satisfying, whether you're baking for others or just yourself. Many store-bought, factory-processed gluten-free baked goods do not meet the high standards we have become used to for taste, flavor and texture in baking, but we can show you that it is possible to be gluten-free, have improved nutrition and still eat tasty foods! Not only can gluten-free baking be delicious, but as an added benefit, our recipes contain ingredients that replace traditional gluten-containing ingredients with even healthier options. Even if you are not consciously avoiding gluten, the recipes in this book are still for you! We will show you how using ancient grain alternatives from many superfoods helps to ensure that your family, friends and guests can truly enjoy what they eat, while benefitting from the nutritional content (without all the elements and additives with long names that we can neither pronounce nor identify).

Baking gluten-free does not require any special skills — it's not complicated or strange. It can be simple and nutritious, tasty and delicious! We've got revamped old favorites as well as new and unique ideas sure to impress anyone you serve them to — including yourself. The results will be wonderful. We have familiar treats such as chocolate cake and classic favorites such as enriched white bread with reduced sugar and fat. Our white bread has been made as close as possible to the gluten-containing version, but we've enhanced it with ancient grains. Our Fluffy White Quinoa Cake (page 82) has improved nutritional value with cooked, pureed quinoa seeds that not only add vitamins and minerals but also reduce the amount of fats and moisture required. We have included healthy recipes such as loaves and granola bars that can be eaten regularly — even daily — as nutritious snacks. So whether you're a gluten-avoider or have an illness that prevents you from eating gluten, these recipes demonstrate that homemade baking made with gluten-free whole foods may be a more delicious option than ever.

If you're not familiar with our books, we'd like to assure you that all of our recipes are repeatedly tested and contain easily sourced ingredients with easy-to-follow instructions. No unusual culinary expertise is required! We will teach you everything you need to know, so enjoy! We are always pleased to read your opinions and feedback at patriciaandcarolyn.com.

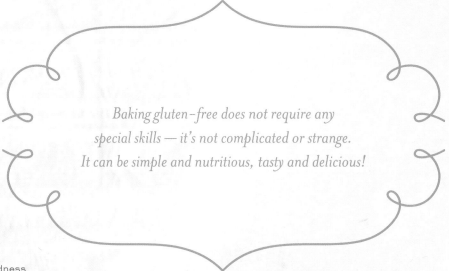

Baking gluten-free does not require any
special skills — it's not complicated or strange.
It can be simple and nutritious, tasty and delicious!

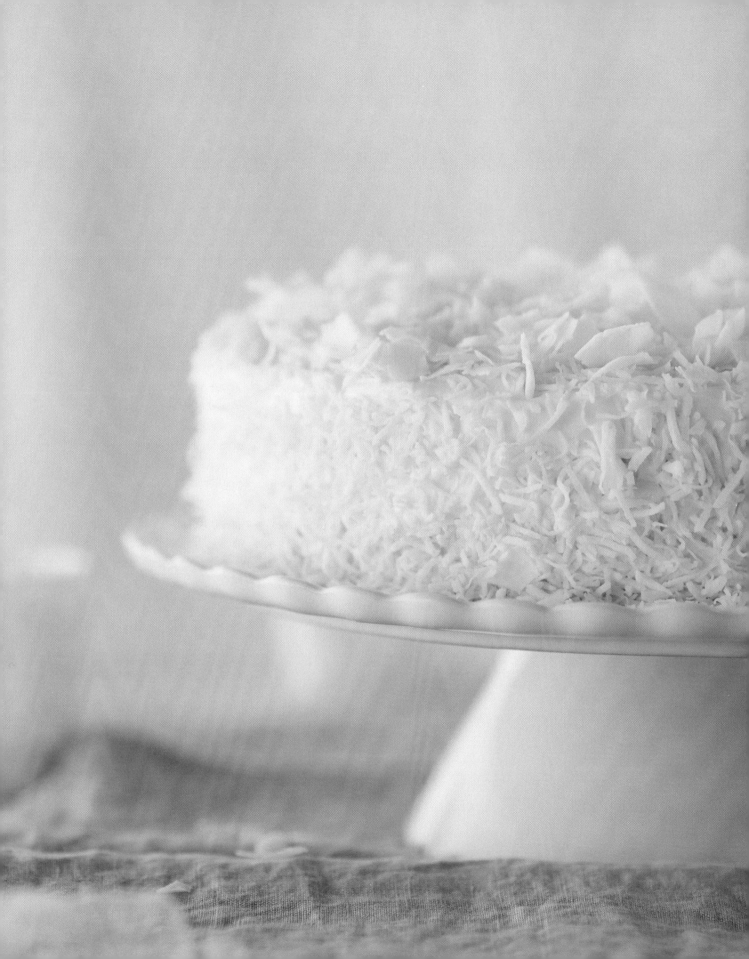

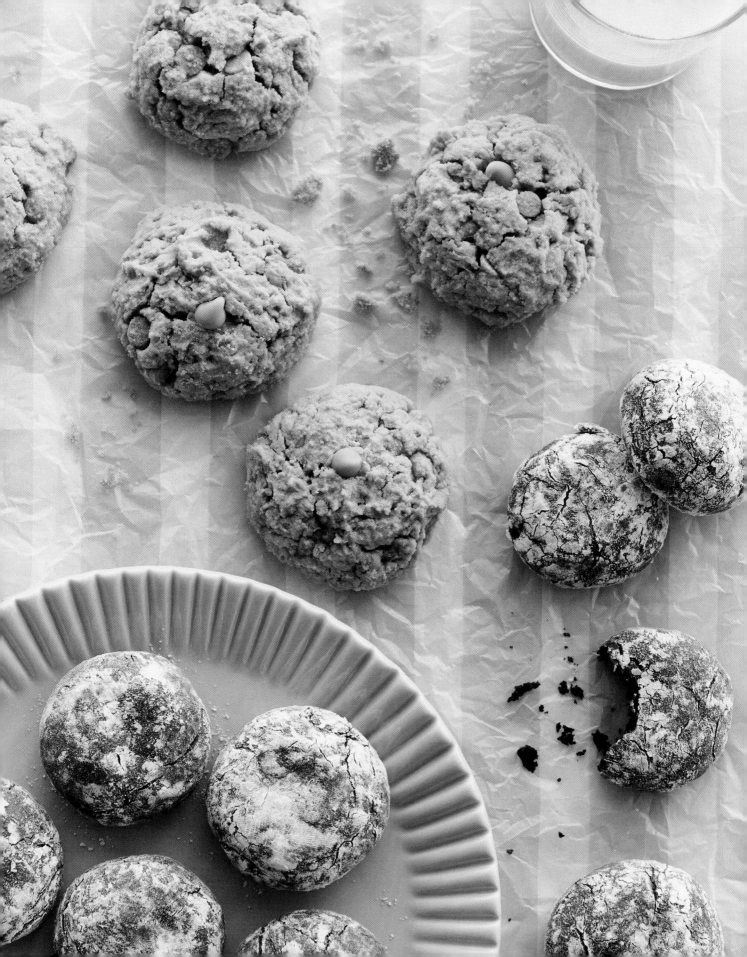

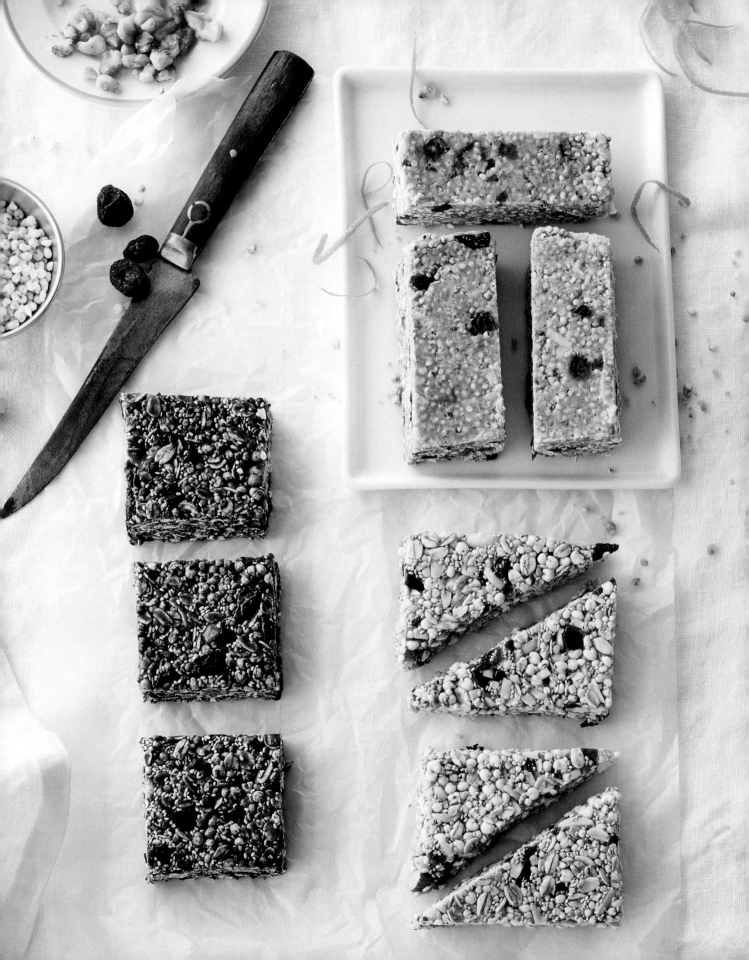

Essentials of Gluten-Free Baking

Tasty and nutritious baking without gluten? Yes! Gluten-free baking doesn't mean you have to settle for chewing on sugar-saturated, cardboard-like cookies or heavy, dense breads. Not in these recipes! We will show you how to make delicious cookies, cakes, pies and more, all without gluten. Sure, there are plenty of store-bought, processed options available, but many of them are severely lacking in nutritional value, never mind flavor and texture.

So why is gluten a problem? Basically, glutens are proteins, some, but not all, of which can cause problems. All grains contain a mixture of proteins, some of them potentially beneficial, some less so. The biggest problem-causing gluten protein currently identified is gliadin, found in wheat, barley and rye. It is known to trigger allergies and digestive issues and is the main culprit behind celiac disease. Research is still needed to confirm if other proteins are equally responsible for reactions or illness, but current information and research suggest that this particular troublemaker is the one to avoid.

Which brings us to the question of what glutens contribute to baking. They're quite helpful in baking, as they bind and provide elasticity, allowing baked goods to hold their shape. They may also alter the fluidity of a batter or dough and can influence rising. However, the reality is that unless the recipe is a dough and needs to be pliable, gluten may not even always be necessary. Quick breads — for example, brownies and pancakes — do not necessarily need gluten, even if it could benefit their structure and texture. Do you recall using any recipes that instruct you not to overmix? Did you ever wonder why? It's so that any gluten present is not activated.

There are actually a wide range of common ingredients that can be used to create delicious, gluten-free baking. That is, baking that is not different in taste and texture from baking that contains gluten. Sometimes there is a loss of moisture in gluten-free baking because of flours and starches that soak up too much liquid. The use of ingredients such as psyllium, flax, chia, liquid honey, pure maple syrup, yogurt, applesauce (and other pureed soft fruits and vegetables), buttermilk and healthy oils helps to alleviate this issue. Cooked ancient grains, such as quinoa, can also help to retain moisture and in some cases reduce how much fat is needed in a recipe.

An increase in the number of accessible, certified gluten-free ingredients (whole, natural and real foods, that is, not packaged foods) on the market means that gluten-free baking is easier and better than ever. In addition to being made into flours, gluten-free seeds and grains can be cooked whole then used in baking, or used as flakes (sliced or rolled grains and seeds) or puffs. In addition, whole, genetically unmodified ingredients such as raisins, cranberries, almonds and other nuts, coconut and cocoa can add enhanced nutrition to your recipes without compromising the final result. This means you can eat gluten-free and healthy, and enjoy your food all at the same time. We always keep in mind that baking is baking, and everything should be eaten in moderation — after all, food is medicine!

GRAIN does not mean GLUTEN!
Traditional grains (cereal grains) are grasses and their
starchy seeds are used as food. Some contain gluten and some
do not. Grains such as corn, oats, sorghum and teff
are examples of grains that do not contain gluten.

Flours and Starches

Flours and starches from seeds and grains can be used as the base for recipes, as thickeners and as part of flour blends. It seems there are many new gluten-free flours being introduced every day. Montina, mesquite, sweet potato, wild rice, pea protein and garfava flour are just a few. All flours have their own characteristics and offer different nutritional profiles. They can all be quite useful in flour blends. For a complete listing of gluten-free flours currently available, see Popular Gluten-Free Ingredients (page 188). In gluten-free baking, you usually have to blend flours to provide the combination of characteristics required to create the proper structure, texture, density and flavor. In many cases, you can make a range of substitutions depending on your personal taste, specific nutritional requirements or even what is available in your supermarket or in your cupboard. However, as with all baking, keep in mind that making changes often means experimenting. Substituting even minor ingredients can produce very different results, possibly affecting flavor, texture, moisture or all of the above.

Starches are important in gluten-free baking, improving the overall crumb, texture and taste, and helping to make baking lighter, softer and more golden. All starches have their own individual characteristics to help enhance the flour used in the recipe. Starches have a tendency to absorb more moisture than regular all-purpose flour. Some of the gluten-free flour blends for sale in stores contain large quantities of starch to ensure your recipes turn out great, but this may come at the expense of the nutritional value. (Our recipes use the least amount of starch and contain the maximum nutritional value possible.) Occasionally, more than one starch is used in a recipe. Starch combining may be done to improve the overall texture and flavor of the baking even further. In gluten-free baking, corn, tapioca and potato starch are a favorite combination for making baked goods lighter and fluffier. Keep in mind that starches do not offer much nutritional value, so we limit the use of large proportions wherever possible, but starches remain invaluable in gluten-free baking.

Maximize freshness by storing flours that are higher in natural oils in the refrigerator. Nut flours; soy, pea and potato flours; brown rice flour and garbanzo, garfava and chickpea flours are less shelf-stable and require refrigeration. If you are unsure, store it in the refrigerator or a cold room. Warm, humid environments can quickly deteriorate flours, making them rancid before their formal expiry date. Many flours and starches can be stored in sealed containers such as wide-mouth containers or glass jars (glass is nonreactive) and kept in a cool, dry place like a dark cupboard. To keep flours even longer, you can store them in the refrigerator or freezer (not in glass, but airtight plastic bags work well).

Sprouted flours? On top of getting a great dose of live, healthy, disease-fighting phytonutrients, you may also like to try gluten-free flours that use sprouted seeds and grains and provide the additional benefit of a partially germinated grain. This provides more nutrients and can improve the digestibility of starches. In short, living enzymes help to ensure great digestion because they help to break down the carbohydrates, proteins and fats that we eat. You can purchase sprouted flours in many of the same stores where you purchase gluten-free, ancient grain flours and organic ingredients.

The flours and starches we use throughout this book include almond flour, amaranth flour, arrowroot starch, brown rice flour, buckwheat flour (light and dark), coconut flour, cornstarch, hazelnut flour, millet flour, oat flour, potato starch, quinoa flour, sorghum flour, sweet rice flour, tapioca starch, teff flour and white rice flour. (For an extended list of gluten-free flours and their properties beyond the ones that we use, see page 188.)

ALMOND FLOUR Made from whole, ground blanched almonds, this flour has a subtle nutty flavor and a dense, finer grind than almond meal (unblanched almonds). It can sometimes be a substitute for oat flour. Nut flours and meals should always be refrigerated. Prolonged exposure to high heat may damage some of the nutrients in nut flours.

AMARANTH FLOUR (SEEDS, FLAKES, PUFFS) This small gluten-free seed from the spinach family can be found in seed, flour, flake and puff forms. It is about the size of a sesame seed and light brown in color. It has a sweet, malty, herbaceous flavor that can be quite dominant in both the seed and flour form. It can become bitter if used in too large a quantity and is considered to be a high-glycemic food. It will cause baking to brown quickly.

ARROWROOT STARCH (FLOUR) This light, white powder extracted from a tropical plant root is used to thicken, especially where transparent color is desired. It smells slightly like anise, but the flavor bakes completely neutral. It absorbs more liquid than other starches and is easy to digest. It makes the best substitute for tapioca starch.

BROWN RICE FLOUR A common flour in gluten-free baking, this is made from milled brown rice grain (hulled, but the rice bran and germ are still intact). It is more fibrous and grainy than white or sweet rice flour and can sometimes create a noticeably coarse texture in baking. It is considered to have a neutral, bland flavor, but is also slightly nutty. It should be stored in the refrigerator. It can be used to thicken, and prevents liquids from separating, especially in frozen or refrigerated baking. It should not be confused with sweet rice flour or rice starch.

BUCKWHEAT FLOUR (LIGHT, DARK, GROATS, FLOUR, FLAKES)
Even though its name contains the word "wheat," it is neither wheat nor related to wheat. It is a gluten-free seed related to rhubarb, green-brown in color and pyramid-shaped. Buckwheat can be bought as seed form (groats), toasted seeds (kasha), flour (light and dark) and flakes. Dark buckwheat flour contains unhulled buckwheat, and light is made from hulled buckwheat (groats). Both flours are high in fiber with a "whole wheat" appearance and have a nutty, earthy aroma, with the dark flour having a

stronger flavor overall. Light buckwheat flour is best for baking, as it has a milder flavor than dark. Dark can be used in recipes where the color is not a factor. Both types of buckwheat flour should be kept in the refrigerator.

COCONUT FLOUR With a light and lovely coconut scent, this flour is made of pure, dried coconut meat that has been ground. It is slightly sweet but can be drying and can make recipes dense because it soaks up much of the moisture. Additional eggs can be used to lighten recipes that use coconut flour. Although from a nut, it is generally considered safe at high temperatures and is higher in fiber and lower in carbohydrates than rice flours are.

CORNSTARCH Sometimes called "corn flour" outside North America, this white starch is extracted from corn and can be useful in building structure in baking and binding. It's not to be confused with cornmeal, which has a much coarser texture. It has a neutral flavor and is widely used in processed gluten-free products and commercial flour blends.

HAZELNUT FLOUR Dried, ground hazelnuts make a powdery flour that has a rich hazelnut aroma often described as nutty and sweet. It has a grainier texture than non-nut flours, but as with other nut flours, it is a lower-carbohydrate option. Nut flours and meals should always be refrigerated. Prolonged exposure to high heat may damage some of the nutrients in nut flours.

MILLET FLOUR (SEEDS, FLAKES, PUFFS) A small, pale, round seed, millet is one of the oldest ancient grains and often regarded as bird seed. Millet flour has a light, mild and neutral flavor, sometimes also noted for its nutty, sweet and dusty taste. It lightens and creates structure in baked goods and can add a creamy yellowish color. It's a great flour for yeast breads, doughs and flatbreads as well as cakes. This gluten-free seed can be found in a variety of forms suitable for baking, including flakes and puffs.

OAT FLOUR (GROATS, FLAKES) Considered an actual grain, oats are still naturally gluten-free. However, unless oats are labeled and certified gluten-free, they can sometimes be contaminated by processing facilities, nearby growing fields or gluten-contaminated soil. Available as groats, steel cut and a variety of flake styles, most oats can be easily ground into oat flour using a good food processor or professional blender. Their neutral flavor and versatility make them a favorite in all types of gluten-free baking, including almost all quick breads. They have a mild binding ability, which helps to build structure and hold together batter, although they should not be used as the sole binding agent in a recipe.

POTATO STARCH Potato starch is made from pressed and peeled raw potatoes. Wet starchy proteins are extracted and then watered down, dehydrated and dried into a powder. It makes a good thickener and is often used as part of a gluten-free flour blend. Potato starch is sometimes referred to as "potato starch flour." Potato starch does not absorb a lot of moisture unless it is heated. It has a moderate binding ability, but helps doughs and batters to rise and lighten, and can make them chewier. It is best used along with tapioca or cornstarch.

QUINOA FLOUR (SEEDS, FLAKES, PUFFS) An ancient grain, gluten-free, superfood seed with a variety of nutritional benefits, quinoa is widely available in multiple forms and is a great asset to gluten-free baking. Quinoa flour is a dense, nutritious flour with a nutty, earthy flavor, which makes it very versatile in a variety of flour blends in all types of baking recipes. Overuse in a blend can result in an overpowering flavor.

SORGHUM FLOUR (GRAINS) Also known as sweet sorghum, this gluten-free grain is a fabulous addition to any gluten-free flour blend. It contains ancient grain, whole-food nutrition that promotes digestion and has a light, nutty yet neutral flavor that works great in most baking recipes. It is often considered to closely resemble the flavor of wheat. It has a dull color and a superfine texture that make it versatile and great for most quick breads.

SWEET RICE FLOUR Ground from short-grain brown or white rice, this is also known as glutinous (sticky) rice (does not contain gluten). It has a higher starch content than plain rice flours and provides great thickening ability. It has a bland, neutral taste and a light color, making it ideal for baking. It's often called "sweet white rice flour," but should not be confused with plain white rice flour (it's not as starchy).

TAPIOCA STARCH (FLOUR) Tapioca starch is the same thing as tapioca flour. It is made from extracting starch from the cassava root. It is neutral and tasteless and may lighten dense breads and cakes when added to flour blends. It may also improve rising when used with yeast, speed browning and make baking chewier. It can be used as a thickening agent and holds together better than other starches do. The closest substitute is cornstarch. Overuse can result in a gummy texture.

TEFF FLOUR (GRAINS) The smallest grain, it offers tremendous nutritional advantages, making it a great addition to flour blends, especially where its dark color is not a concern. Its flavor is slightly sour and nutty. Darker versions of the flour have more of a molasses flavor and the taste of lighter teff flour is often compared to that of hazelnut flour. The flavor of teff flour can overpower if too much is used or if no complementary or competing flavors are included. It is mucilaginous (gel-like) when combined with water.

WHITE RICE FLOUR Made from milled long- or medium-grain or polished white rice, it is also referred to as simply "rice flour." A popular and widely available gluten-free flour, white rice flour has a neutral taste, a neutral color and some thickening ability. It can sometimes make the texture of baked goods grainy. It is not to be confused with sweet rice flour, brown rice flour or rice starch.

Flour Blends

Although you can buy a variety of pre-formulated gluten-free flour blends in stores, we highly recommend you make your own. Store-bought blends are mostly made up of starches, if not completely of starch. The results can be inconsistent: some may not work well at all or they may offer little to no nutrition, or a combination of these things. Instead, we recommend you keep a variety of your own gluten-free flours on hand so you can easily make your own blends. This gives you control over the taste, texture and nutrition in your recipes. Generally, for most baking, you can use 25%–30% of any one flour as part of a blend. Some recipes can handle more than that. For example, brownies or cookies may be able to use 100% of one particular flour. The type of baking recipe (bread, cookie, cake, pastry, etc.) and its characteristics (complementing flavors, texture) really determine the proportions of flour blends you can use more than the type of flour determines how much you can use of it. There are many nutritious, gluten-free flours readily available, allowing you to make your own flour blends simply and quickly. Blending flours not only incorporates various nutritional profiles but also combines flavor affinities and characteristics for great baking results. Blending may improve flavor, helping to neutralize any dominating tastes and allowing for increased baking versatility. In this book, we have used certain ancient grain flours where their specific baking characteristics and flavor lend themselves to particular recipes.

If you usually prefer store-bought flour blends to save time, we recommend instead that you choose your favorite recipes and premix the dry ingredients (using the homemade flour blends in our recipes) then place them in resealable bags, labeled and dated, to freeze until needed.

When you make your own combinations you can also enhance the nutritional value of a recipe. For instance, if you want to make your recipe a complete protein and are using millet flour (which lacks a high enough level of the amino acid lysine to be considered a complete protein on its own), adding some amaranth flour (high in lysine) will complete the protein requirements of the recipe's nutritional profile. Adding any ancient grains that are complete proteins (that is, they contain adequate levels of lysine) would also make this a complete protein.

Blends may assist with specific dietary restrictions. For instance, some gluten-free flours are lower glycemic than others; higher in dietary fiber, calcium, essential fatty acids, antioxidants and B complex vitamins; complete proteins or just easier to digest than others. Some cook quicker than others, increase volume in baking or provide or absorb more moisture.

There are recipes where using a single flour can be effective — brownies, pancakes and crêpes are a few examples. However, even these recipes can be made even better with a flour blend. In general, blends of various gluten-free flours are used to ensure success.

Grinding Your Own Flours

Generally, all seeds and grains (whole or flaked) can be made into flour. Flour is best made from whole seed, which contains the most nutritional integrity. Milling at home can be an economical and healthy way of using gluten-free flours. For smaller amounts, grinding can be done with a simple mortar and pestle. For larger amounts, a coffee grinder, seed mill or good blender can be used. But use caution when using flour grinders! Depending on the grinder, a heavier oil content in some seeds or grains can ruin an expensive grinder. Be sure to check your grinder's user manual. And consider keeping your coffee grinder only for grinding flour, to avoid taste contamination.

Store-bought milled flour is more finely ground, and when you grind at home the results will differ depending on the appliance used. A coffee grinder or blender may result in a grind closer to a "meal," producing a coarser flour. This may lead to a heavier density in your recipes. Extra grinding may help to create a finer grind. And a quality professional blender may provide a finer grind.

One of the easiest flours to make yourself is oat flour. You simply grind the oat flakes in a blender until you have a fine grind. It is more difficult to grind flours from seeds, nuts, beans and legumes, which are richer in oils. When you purchase many of these flours already ground, however, the seeds, beans or nuts will have been either partially or wholly defatted. This ensures that a usable, dry, powdery flour results from the grind, instead of a butter or creamy, wet substance that cannot be used as flour.

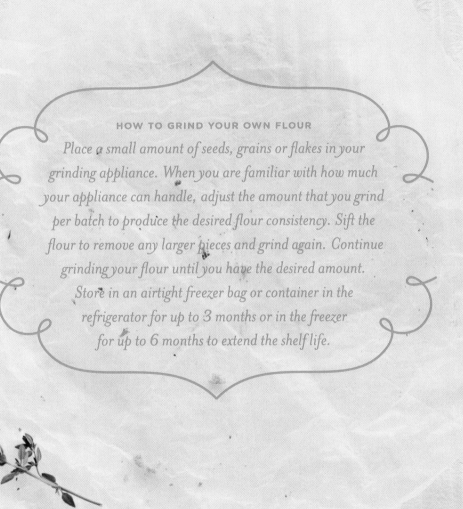

HOW TO GRIND YOUR OWN FLOUR

Place a small amount of seeds, grains or flakes in your grinding appliance. When you are familiar with how much your appliance can handle, adjust the amount that you grind per batch to produce the desired flour consistency. Sift the flour to remove any larger pieces and grind again. Continue grinding your flour until you have the desired amount. Store in an airtight freezer bag or container in the refrigerator for up to 3 months or in the freezer for up to 6 months to extend the shelf life.

Weighing and Measuring Flours

Weighing flours is a secret of the pros. It can help improve the accuracy in gluten-free baking, ensuring your recipes turn out exactly as you want them to — consistently. In this book, we have already provided you with accurate amounts in cups and volume options (mL), but weighing flours can be especially important if you are making substitutions with other gluten-free flours or converting any of your old favorite gluten-containing recipes into gluten-free. Gluten-free flours can be heavier or lighter than the conventional, gluten-containing versions, and when you weigh them, you may find you require less or more than the conventional flours your recipes call for. When measuring your gluten-free flour into cups, stir the flour in its container, then lightly spoon the flour into the measuring cup over a piece of parchment. Heap the flour, but avoid tapping, shaking or packing it. Carefully level the flour with a flat edge (a knife is ideal) and let the excess fall onto the parchment. Pour the excess back into the storage container. Measuring the flour out this way will help to ensure that your recipes turn out successfully.

The ancient grain, gluten-free flours that we use in this book are those that we feel work the best for baking, are the most widely accessible and also offer some increased nutrition. The starches we use are in the smallest quantities possible and are only used where they are essential to a specific recipe's outcome.

WEIGH IN

If you're substituting ingredients or creating your own recipes, weighing is a more accurate method of measuring and can be helpful in ensuring your gluten-free recipes turn out well. If you don't want to weigh (or if you don't have kitchen scales), you can still bake successfully by carefully measuring gluten-free flours and ingredients (do not tap or pack ingredients in measuring cups, etc.). In this book, we have done the measuring work for you, making it easy for you to continue using conventional, accessible baking methods that everyone is used to.

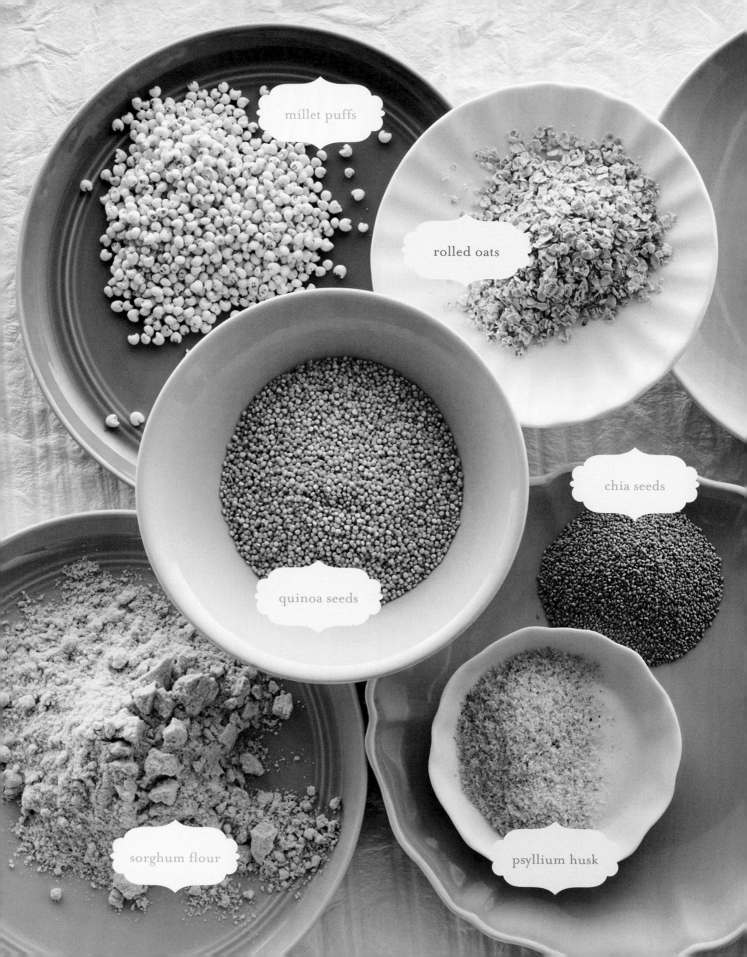

millet puffs

rolled oats

chia seeds

quinoa seeds

sorghum flour

psyllium husk

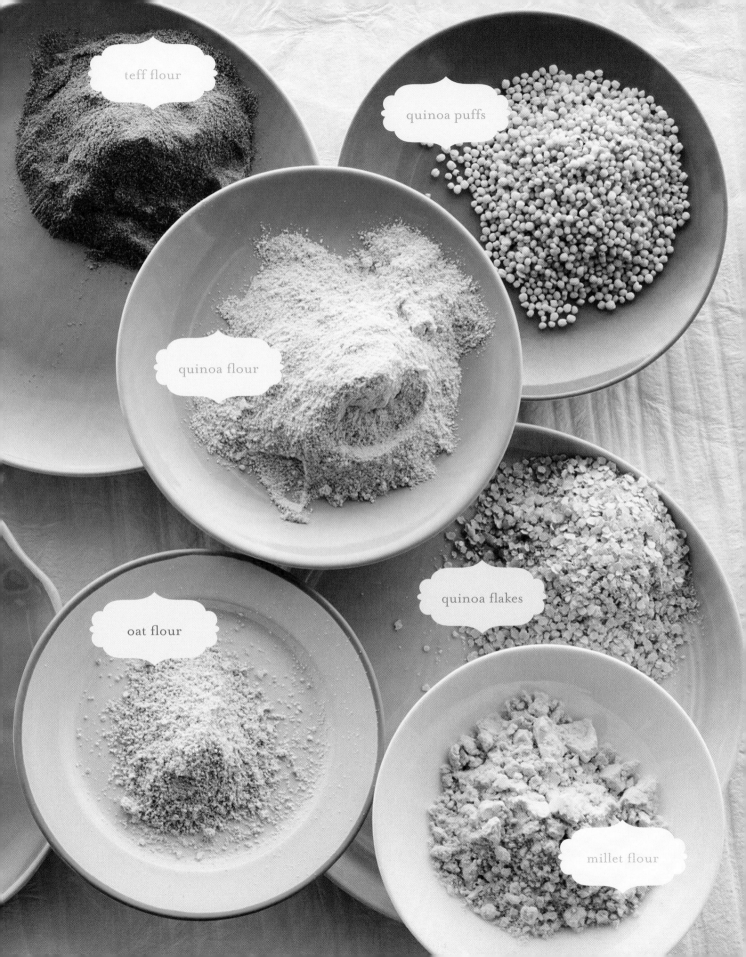

Binders and Stabilizers

Conventional baking recipes rely on gluten to bind and hold together many different types of baked goods. Although not always necessary, some type of alternative binder is often required. Referred to as thickeners, binders or stabilizers, they can be essential in recipes that do not contain gluten. They help to hold ingredients together, reduce crumbling and add volume to gluten-free baking, especially doughs. Chia (ground or whole), ground flax seeds and psyllium husks can make excellent gels or binders to make up for the absence of gluten. You may have one that you prefer or that works best for your digestion or personal dietary preferences. Guar and xanthan gums behave similarly to each other.

Guar gum originates from legumes and xanthan gum is derived from corn. Overuse of either can make baked goods too heavy and dense. Xanthan gum holds together mixtures such as pastry and can mimic the "spring" of bread. Guar gum is a good alternative to xanthan gum if you have corn allergies, but it is very high in fiber and can cause stomach upset, especially if you are sensitive to it and if it is not used sparingly. The general rule is to add approximately 1 teaspoon (5 mL) of guar or xanthan gum for every 1 cup (250 mL) of gluten-free flour in recipes that don't require much leavening. For recipes that require a lot of leavening, you can expect to increase this amount to approximately 1 ½ teaspoons (7 mL) of guar or xanthan gum for every 1 cup (250 mL) of gluten-free flour, but it will vary according to the recipe.

If you prefer not to use guar or xanthan gum, in many cases you can use psyllium husks, eggs, chia or ground flax seeds instead. And they bring an additional benefit. Not only do each of them help to bind the batter or dough, they also provide some additional nutrition, where guar and xanthan gums may not.

Chia and flax can also be used to replace up to 25% of all fats, such as butter, in a recipe, although neither is strong enough to act alone as a binder for most doughs or yeast breads. Simply leaving out guar or xanthan gum without adding something else to bind the mixture can result in a final product that is too wet. Psyllium, chia or flax can help absorb additional moisture. Psyllium especially can help make doughs more flexible and strong.

Vegan alternatives to traditional binders (such as eggs) include gelatin, tofu and agar agar (seaweed powder), as well as bananas and other soft fruit. Thickening agents also include sweet rice flour, rice starch, arrowroot starch, tapioca starch (flour), potato starch and teff grains, which have mucilaginous properties. The binders and thickeners you choose to use will depend on personal preference, dietary requirements and market availability. Each may be used in slightly different quantities depending on the type of recipe you use them in. As you do more gluten-free baking and become more confident, you'll find you develop a feel for which substitutes work best for you and your recipes.

No need to knead?

If there is no gluten required in the recipe you are preparing (it's not a dough, for instance) then there is no need to work the dough as you would in a gluten-containing recipe. Some of our doughs or batters seem to work best with simply a few minutes of mixing to ensure all the ingredients are incorporated.

The binders and stabilizers we use throughout this book are chia, eggs, psyllium husks and xanthan gum.

CHIA (SEEDS, GROUND) Chia is one of nature's great plant sources of omega-3s. These gluten-free seeds can be used whole or ground to enhance moisture retention, crumb and texture in cooking (not to mention nutritional value!). The mucilaginous properties of chia make it a good alternative for binding in baking, used in a proportion of 25%–50% of fat or egg. (In general, that means using 1 teaspoon/5 mL of ground chia or chia seeds in ¼ cup/60 mL of water to replace ¼ cup/60 mL of butter or fat or one egg.) It helps breads to be softer, holds moisture and is thought to act as a natural preservative. It does not bind strongly enough to be used on its own as a binder for doughs and yeast breads, though.

EGGS Eggs are a natural binder, leavener and fat used in conventional baking. Beaten eggs (especially whites) also help to add volume and rising by holding air bubbles inside the batter. Room-temperature eggs help to create even more volume. If you are vegan or have allergies, you can use one of many substitutes, including chia, flax and psyllium, depending on the recipe.

PSYLLIUM HUSKS The strongest of the natural binders, psyllium husks, whole or ground, lend enough strength to work well in doughs and yeast breads where other natural binders may fail. Psyllium husks can be used as the sole binder in many recipes.

XANTHAN GUM This has no real nutritional value, but it is the most common binder, used to thicken and add volume to baked goods.

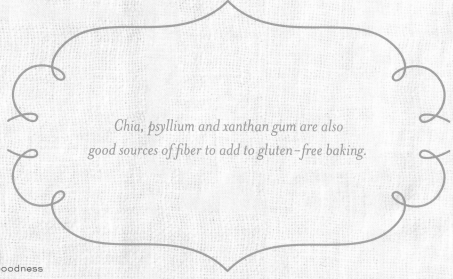

*Chia, psyllium and xanthan gum are also
good sources of fiber to add to gluten-free baking.*

Leavening Agents

Leavening agents, or leaveners, help to provide volume and shape and to create texture in baking. When baking gluten-free, using exact amounts of these ingredients can be key to your success. We use baking powder, baking soda, cream of tartar and yeast to leaven doughs and breads and promote rising.

BAKING POWDER A *chemical* leavener, this is a powdered leavening agent that usually contains a mixture of baking soda and a weaker acid such as cream of tartar and a starch to prevent lumps. When combined with moisture, it will lighten and add volume to baking by releasing gases that form air inside the dough or batter. It's used in quick breads. As conventional baking powder may contain gluten, it is important to purchase brands specifically labeled gluten-free. Or you can easily make your own gluten-free baking powder. Just mix 1 teaspoon (5 mL) of baking soda with 2 teaspoons (10 mL) of cream of tartar.

BAKING SODA (SODIUM BICARBONATE) A *chemical* leavener, household baking soda releases gases if combined with an acid and moisture. It adds air that helps to rise and add volume to baking. It is used in quick breads. As conventional baking soda may contain gluten, it is important to purchase brands specifically labeled gluten-free.

CREAM OF TARTAR An acid that is often used to activate baking soda (along with moisture). It helps to strengthen as well as add and maintain volume in baking.

YEAST A *biological* leavener, yeast releases gases when moisture and carbohydrates are added and it ferments. It requires more time to rise (warmth helps) and so needs a strong dough or batter to hold the gas in longer. Yeast encourages rising but may influence the taste of the baked product, so use only as much as required.

If you are new to gluten-free baking, we suggest that you follow our recipes exactly as written, without making substitutions, to achieve the best possible results. It can be expensive and time-consuming to have recipes fail, so we recommend that you wait until you are more familiar with gluten-free baking before you experiment and play with the recipes. Ensure you are always using ingredients labeled gluten-free, even where making substitutions.

For all flours, starches, binders and leaveners used in this book, we try to use the ingredients that offer the most nutritional value first. Keep in mind that there are pros and cons about using many gluten-free ingredients. Know what your options are and make choices based on what is right for you. Use what works for your dietary restrictions and preferences, and what you have access to in your local market.

Sweeteners

In our recipes we use mostly organic cane sugar, honey, pure maple syrup and lightly packed brown sugar. The type of sugar used in baking is critical, as it can significantly impact the finished product. Sugar often has a strong influence on structure, so our choices of sweeteners are specific to each recipe. Please note this before you attempt to make substitutions with sweeteners.

There is currently not enough scientific evidence about the health benefits of sweeteners such as agave, coconut sugar and other trends in sugar alternatives for us to consistently promote their use, whether they claim to be better-for-you or sustainable options. Until we have good, solid evidence about their health benefits and other properties, we'll be sticking to our current choice of traditional sweeteners in baking. As conscious consumers, we recommend you make the best choice for yourself. Remember, if it's baking, it likely contains some sweetener and should be eaten in moderation anyway. It's a treat!

Where possible, we recommend the use of honey, pure maple syrup, organic cane sugar, Sucanat and organic muscovado, Demerara or turbinado sugar instead of more highly processed sugars. Where organic cane sugar is listed in the ingredients you may use regular white sugar. You may also swap lightly packed brown sugar for muscovado sugar. However, muscovado contains more moisture than regular brown sugar, so be sure to reduce the overall moisture in the recipe by at least 1 tablespoon (15 mL). Use caution if choosing Sucanat, Demerara or turbinado sugars, as they can be coarse and may require some grinding prior to being measured and added to your recipe. Using coarse sugars without grinding them first may make for uneven blending or undissolved patches, spots or blotches in your doughs and batters. Coconut sugar and Sucanat may work in some recipes, but may change the structure, flavor and texture of your baking and, in fact, may not work well. If you decide to experiment with substitutes, expect that these sweeteners may dramatically change the outcome of your recipe. You will notice our choice of sweeteners varies throughout the book. This is because our primary goal is to design these gluten-free recipes to be as close in taste, texture and flavor to what you'd expect from the popular, familiar versions found in the traditional North American diet. In some cases, using a sweetener that has a higher moisture content, such as liquid honey or syrup, can too adversely impact structure or crumb, where organic cane sugar would provide more stability. Keep in mind that using syrups, liquid honey, agave and other high-moisture sweeteners can not only change the outcome of the recipe, but also dramatically shorten the shelf life of your finished baked goods. These are our sweeteners of choice:

CANE SUGAR (ORGANIC) Organic, whole and natural sugar cane juice is evaporated and dried. This works well as a replacement for white granulated sugar in baking recipes.

COCONUT SUGAR Sap is extracted from coconut palm trees then cooked, dehydrated and crystallized. It is a granular sugar, but often the crystals are large, requiring additional grinding at home. Not to be confused with palm sugar.

DEMERARA SUGAR A less-refined, yellow-colored cane sugar made from pressed sugar cane. This may have a coarser texture than granulated and require additional grinding, and it can be expensive. It is often referred to as "raw sugar."

HONEY Nectar from flowers is collected, broken down and stored by bees. The water evaporates in the comb shapes of the hive, making a thick syrup. This liquid syrup works well as a sweetener in some recipes, but its higher moisture content reduces the shelf-life of baked goods, so its use in baking may be limited to selected recipes.

MAPLE SYRUP (PURE) Sap from maple trees is extracted, then cooked to evaporate the water. This liquid syrup works well as a sweetener in some recipes, but its higher moisture content reduces the shelf-life of baked goods, so its use in baking may be limited to selected recipes.

MUSCOVADO SUGAR A less-refined sugar made from dehydrated sugar cane juice, this contains more molasses than other sugars. It is a granular sugar with a darker color and a sticky consistency, but it can be used in place of brown sugar in many cases. Its slightly higher moisture content (compared to regular brown sugar) may necessitate moisture reductions elsewhere in baking recipes.

SUCANAT A brand name of an unrefined cane sugar. Its darker appearance comes from the molasses content. It may be coarse and require additional grinding.

TURBINADO SUGAR A less-refined sugar made from dehydrated sugar cane juice. It's often referred to as "raw sugar," and may have a coarser texture and require additional grinding.

GRINDING SUCANAT SUGAR

Place coarse Sucanat sugar in a coffee grinder and grind until it resembles a fine powder.

Dairy

Because some celiacs also develop a protein allergy that may result in an intolerance to dairy, you may choose to use alternatives if celiac disease is a consideration.

Coconut milk, soy milk, rice milk, hemp and almond milk (and a variety of other nut milks) are good substitutions. Keep in mind that recipe results may vary. You can also make gluten-free milks from ancient grains and seeds. If you can't find gluten-free sour cream, plain yogurt is generally a good alternative. Need to substitute buttermilk or don't have any on hand? To make ½ cup (125 mL), use a scant ½ cup (125 mL) of regular milk or dairy-free milk and add ½ tablespoon (7.5 mL) of white vinegar or lemon juice. Let rest for about 5 minutes, then use. (Note that you can't use this substitution in all recipes. In recipes that use buttermilk, we'll let you know if this substitute is an option.) If you want to use dairy-free milk, we find almond or organic soy works best. Other milks may produce different, unexpected results. If dairy-free milk is an option for a recipe, you'll see it listed in the ingredients.

Oils, Fats and Eggs

In many cases, our baking recipes use a standard favorite: butter. Real butter is natural, not manufactured in a laboratory, and your body knows how to deal with it when you eat it. It is simply made from natural ingredients and you can even make it in your own kitchen. Nut butters are an alternative, but their distinctive tastes and textures will affect the recipe, so they are best used only when indicated. Virgin organic coconut oil (also sometimes called "raw" coconut oil) is a great option along with organic palm oil, unrefined olive oil or grapeseed oil. If using coconut oil, keep in mind that like other oils, the "refined" type is different from "virgin" in terms of both flavor and nutritional properties. For instance, refined oil may not have the coconut flavor of virgin coconut oil, which may be ideal in some recipes, but may also not have the nutritional properties that virgin coconut oil has. Decide what you want to use and make your own choice. To substitute eggs, you can use a powdered egg substitute; binders such as psyllium husk, ground flax and chia can work similarly. How much to substitute? That varies according to the recipe, so it's impossible to offer a general guideline. Luckily, there are many online tools to help you make decisions.

Baking Equipment Essentials

Some pieces of kitchen equipment are invaluable in gluten-free baking.

OVEN THERMOMETER Some oven thermostats can be off by significant amounts. Having an oven thermometer helps you to keep an eye on the temperature and so produce properly baked goods. If you are experiencing repeated failures, this could help.

INSTANT READ THERMOMETER This is essential for successfully making a loaf, bread or buns. It can be very difficult to determine the level of doneness of baked goods based on time or color or by tapping the bread. Using an instant read thermometer ensures the center is baked. Loaves, breads and buns should read between 205°F and 207°F (105–110°C) before you remove them from the oven.

STAND MIXER This is an important item on your equipment list. Its ease and dependability will have you saving time and energy. Being able to use a paddle, whisk or dough hook where required is invaluable in the gluten-free kitchen. A hand mixer is not suitable for heavier doughs and strong hand kneading may not be sufficient. The stand mixer is a worthy investment.

SILICONE SPATULA This works fabulously in removing all the dough you worked so hard to pay for and make.

STAINLESS STEEL SPRING ACTION SCOOPS These are ideal for scooping out doughs and batters in premeasured amounts. Most of all, they keep your hands clean and things tidy. The best sizes are ½ oz (1 Tbsp/15 mL) and 1 oz (2 Tbsp/30 mL) for things like cookies, and 2 oz (¼ cup/60 mL) for muffins, buns and cupcakes.

BAKING SHEETS AND PANS Baking sheets that fit your oven for cookies and tarts as well as standard cake pans are essential. Standard cake pans are 9-inch (2.5 L) square or round, 8-inch (2 L) square or round, 13- × 9-inch (3 L), 9- × 5-inch (2 L) loaf pans, springform and Bundt pans. Muffin tins and mini-muffin tins are invaluable for cupcakes, muffins and other treats that bake in individual serving sizes. For standard-sized pies that serve 8 to 10, you'll need 10-inch (25 cm) pie plates.

SAUCEPANS You will need saucepans for melting ingredients such as butter, oils, syrups and chocolate, and for making sauces.

PARCHMENT Parchment paper is invaluable in baking. It helps to provide even browning on the bottom of cookies or cakes, makes for easy removal from pans and — possibly its most important benefit — prevents any metals from the baking pans from leaching into your baking.

BLENDERS, FLOUR GRINDERS OR COFFEE GRINDERS Blenders and grinders can be helpful tools for making your own fresh flours quickly and easily from seeds and grains. Even if you buy most of your gluten-free flours pre-ground, grinders can prove to be essential tools for simply grinding oat flakes into flour. While most blenders may successfully grind flakes to the proper texture to make a baking flour, many will not produce a fine enough, usable grind from other grains and seeds. For this reason you may require a standard grinder for grinding other seeds and grains into flour, but you must be aware of the oil content! Too much oil can damage an expensive grinder beyond repair.

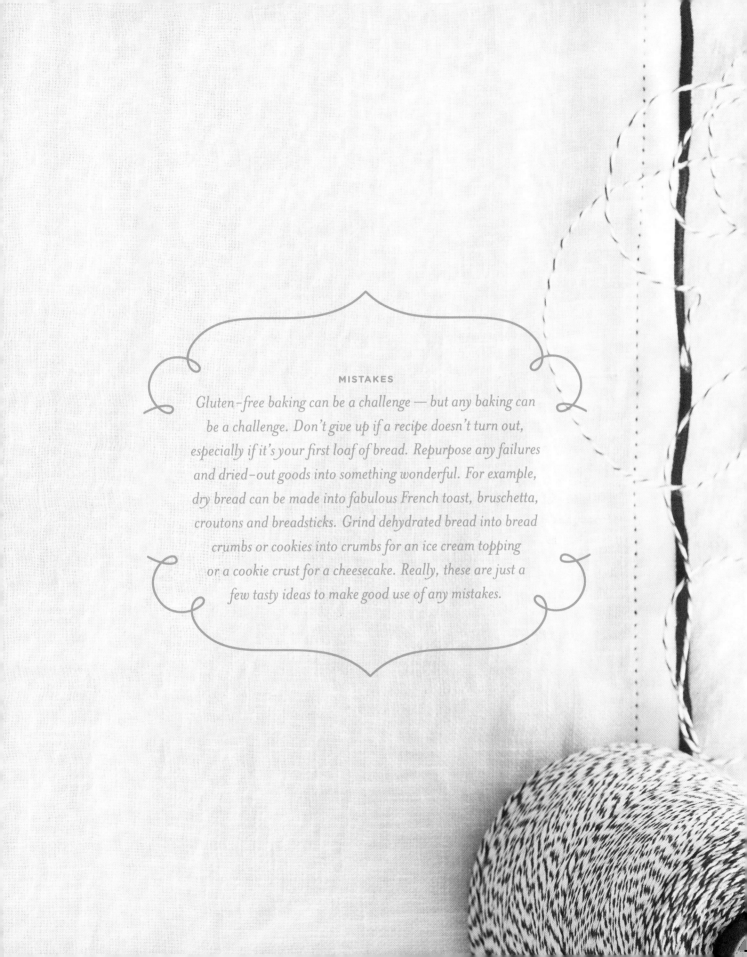

MISTAKES

Gluten-free baking can be a challenge — but any baking can be a challenge. Don't give up if a recipe doesn't turn out, especially if it's your first loaf of bread. Repurpose any failures and dried-out goods into something wonderful. For example, dry bread can be made into fabulous French toast, bruschetta, croutons and breadsticks. Grind dehydrated bread into bread crumbs or cookies into crumbs for an ice cream topping or a cookie crust for a cheesecake. Really, these are just a few tasty ideas to make good use of any mistakes.

Baking Tips

Many of the factors that affect regular baking will affect gluten-free
baking, including, but not limited to, type of pans or bakeware
used; altitude, climate and humidity; substituted ingredients
and ambient (room) temperature. And remember that many
ovens do not heat evenly. Adjust your bake times according to
the quirks of your oven.

RISING AND YEAST BREADS

It is essential that yeast breads rise in a draft-free
environment. Any enclosed area such as an empty, slightly
warm oven, cupboard or other contained space is ideal for
rising as long as it is warm. Many yeast breads traditionally
require gluten to turn out as expected. Yeast bread recipes that
include doughs, pizza doughs, bread and buns will require a binder of
some sort. Psyllium husks, chia seeds or xanthan or guar gum are the usual
choices; all work differently and require tweaking your recipes. Experiment
and use what you choose. And note that using room-temperature eggs and
milk helps to give baking better volume, so if you are making bread,
a fluffy cake or a soufflé, this is the way to go.

FLAKY PASTRY

The secret to flaky pastry is cold ingredients and tools. If your baked pastry is
tough, it could be that there was too much water in the dough. If you have to
increase the moisture because your pastry dough seems too dry, an egg yolk is
a good alternative to water or milk. The fat in pastry helps to keep it tender,
so an egg yolk is a suitable addition. Using cold tools will help (a cold pie
plate helps reduce crust shrinkage) and handling the mixture as little
as possible will ensure it doesn't become too heavy.

ACCURATE MEASURING

It is often better to measure by weight when baking gluten-free (see page xxx for more on this), as all flours measure slightly differently. Flours that are finer may be denser and 1 cup (250 mL) of one particular flour may not be equivalent to 1 cup of another. When using your own substitutions, experiment carefully and keep in mind that your recipes will get better with trial and error.

BAKEWARE

Always watch your baking instead of slavishly adhering to the recommended temperature and baking duration. Goods baked in glass bakeware tend to bake faster (brown quicker) than those in metal pans. Darkened metal will also do the same. Size matters! If you are substituting pan size, keep in mind that the results may be affected. Also, always use the center rack in your oven, unless the recipe specifies otherwise. This will ensure even, thorough baking. Removing your baking from the pans as soon as it's cool enough to do so is critical to prevent the bottom from becoming mushy (depending on the recipe, of course).

ALTITUDE

If you are baking at altitudes of 3,500 feet (1,067 meters) and higher, it is recommended that you slightly reduce the amount of liquid you use (depends on what altitude you are at) and increase baking temperatures by at least 25°F (14°C). Also, baking times may have to be extended. You can find many online resources and guides to help with altitude issues.

HUMIDITY

In humid climates it is recommended to use a tablespoon or two (15–30 mL) less of liquid (this includes things like honey, applesauce, yogurt, etc.) in your recipe. If your kitchen is too humid, take care when removing baked goods, especially gluten-free doughs, from the oven, as they can quickly fall in very humid environments.

STORAGE

Storing your gluten-free baked goods properly is critical in maintaining freshness, as they usually contain more moisture than conventional baking. Specifically, those ingredients that we use as binders also help to retain water. This means that the shelf-life of baking may ultimately be shorter. Airtight containers and refrigeration help to increase and extend freshness.

Gluten-Free Baking Myths

You can't benefit from eating gluten-free

Untrue! Even if you do not have celiac disease, intolerances, allergies or sensitivities, it may be beneficial to eat gluten-free. While we don't necessarily recommend you go completely gluten-free if you don't have to (unless you have a private chef who can ensure that all your meals are sufficiently nutritious), there may be other reasons you choose to be gluten-free or can benefit from eating gluten-free. Research demonstrates that eating gluten-free can enhance athletic performance. The body's natural response to gluten is inflammation in the intestine that can inhibit proper and efficient nutrient absorption, which in turn affects many physiological responses in the body, including reflexes, muscle response, physical endurance, stamina, muscle repair and energy recovery. Eating gluten-free is a choice for some athletes, some of whom are choosing it as their overall lifestyle, while others choose to eat gluten-free at specific times, before and after training or competition. Many of these same athletes swear by the gluten-free approach to eating and claim it increases their performance remarkably. Steve Nash, two-time NBA MVP and seven-time NBA All-Star, and Novak Djokovic, currently one of the top-ranked tennis players in the world and six-time Grand Slam ATP tennis champion, are two examples of elite athletes who eat gluten-free. Most health professionals discourage individuals from eating completely gluten-free or self-diagnosing gluten intolerance because, for the majority, it can lead to poor dietary habits if all aspects are not clearly understood and the proper eating regime is not followed. In some cases, those who make the choice to eat gluten-free are consuming highly processed gluten-free products from store shelves, many of which are laden with sugars and fats and offer inferior nutrition because the products' intention is to be gluten-free, not necessarily to offer nutritional value. Remember the popular food marketing that encouraged everyone to avoid carbohydrates? Did we all remember that the brain absolutely requires carbohydrates to function? With the proper information we can choose the right carbohydrates. To eat well, you need to eat the foodstuffs your body needs to work properly! Don't avoid foods your body needs without proper knowledge or because of fads or fad diets. Be aware. Always speak with a doctor or a health professional before making major changes to your diet.

You will lose weight if you eat gluten-free

This is considered to be a myth because most people who decide
to eat gluten-free make poor alternative food choices. Over-
processed store-bought gluten-free foods often provide little
to no nutrition, contain less protein and may be higher in
fat and sugar, resulting in more damage than good to your
body. On the other hand, if you make healthy, gluten-free
food choices, your circumstances may be different. Eating
a variety of fresh, nutritious, whole foods and vegetables
instead of processed, shelved goods can certainly be of
benefit. Swapping out baking that has inferior nutritional
value with better gluten-free ingredients can also benefit your
body. Always read labels on packages closely. Our goal in this
book is to show you how to transform recipes you may already
be eating that contain gluten into gluten-free alternatives that
provide improved nutritional value and are therefore a healthier
and overall better baking option for you! Just remember: it's still
baking and should be eaten in moderation.

Baking gluten-free is too difficult

Gluten-free baking is not difficult. It just takes a bit of adjustment and
maybe experimenting in the kitchen. Some gluten-free ingredients, such as
ancient grains, offer even better nutritional value than conventional baking
ingredients, and are just as easy to find and use.

Gluten-free baking is inferior in taste, texture and nutrition

We refuse to make our gluten-free baking with large amounts of nutritionally inferior ingredients! We will show you how to bake delicious treats using nutritious gluten-free ingredients. Baking that tastes, looks and smells exactly like you'd expect baking to — but with healthy aspects!

Gluten-free means low calorie

All food (even if you eat cardboard) contains calories, and unfortunately gluten-free does not guarantee low calorie. You simply must choose your types of calories wisely. Remember, not all calories are created equal! Without getting into too much (confusing) detail, at a molecular level, different calories are metabolized differently according to their food source. In our recipes we aim to use ingredients that can provide the best nutrition and great recipe results. Choose ingredients that provide the best nutritional value and meet your specific dietary requirements. And keep in mind that no one advises you to gorge on baking or eat it for every meal. It should always be considered a treat.

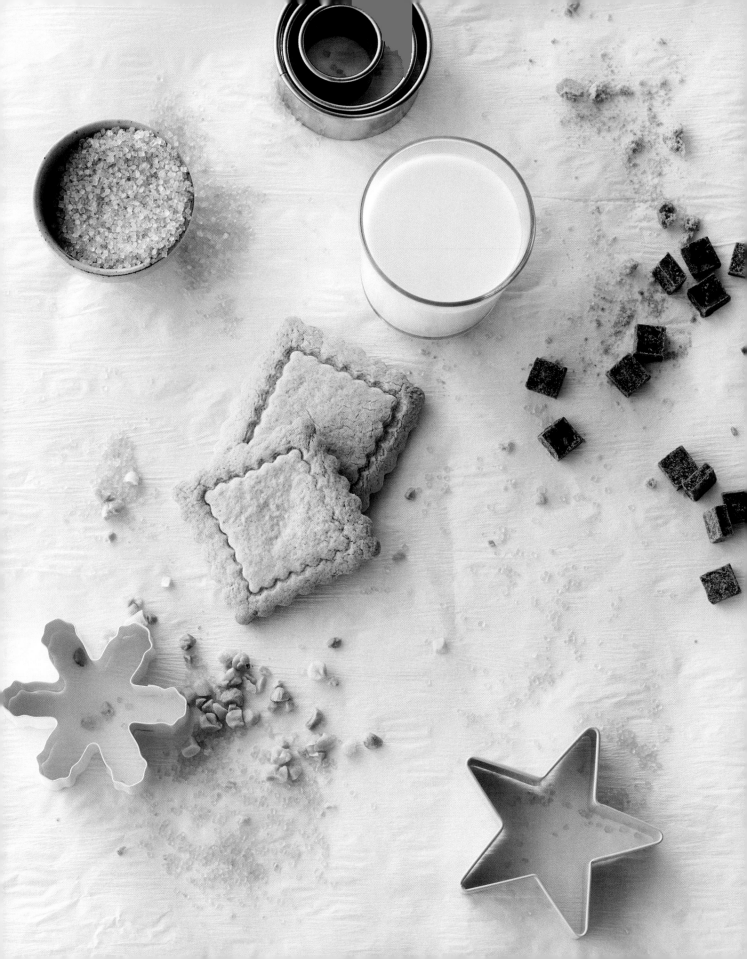

Cookies, Bars and Squares

Carrot Butterscotch Cookies   4

Chewy Raisin Oatmeal
Chia Cookies   6

Oat, Strawberry and Cream Cheese
Thumbprint Cookies   7

Monster Oat Chia Cookies   8

Chocolate Whirl Cookies   9

Peanut Butter Chocolate
Chunk Cookies   11

Mocha Crinkle Cookies   12

Ginger Squash
Molasses Cookies   15

Triple Chocolate
Coconut Chia Cookies   16

Salted Caramel Pecan
Shortbread Bites   17

Oat Fig Newtons   18

Chocolate Whoopie Pies   21

Mint Matcha Morsels   22

Double Chocolate
Sorghum and Teff Biscotti   23

Citrus Sorghum
and Oat Biscotti   24

Cranberry Almond Energy Bites   26

Carrot Apricot Squares   27

Apricot, Walnut and
Pine Nut Granola Bars   29

Apple Raisin Oat Squares   30

Hawaiian Oat Squares   31

White Chocolate, Orange
and Nut Butter Quinoa Squares   32

Chocolate Fruit and Nut Chia
Squares   34

Chocolate, Walnut
and Prune Millet Quinoa Squares   35

Cranberry Lemon Millet
Quinoa Squares   36

Espresso Cookie Bars with
Honey Marshmallow Meringue   38

Milk Chocolate and
Orange Blondies   39

Praline Cheesecake Blondies   40

Chocolate Hazelnut Brownies   41

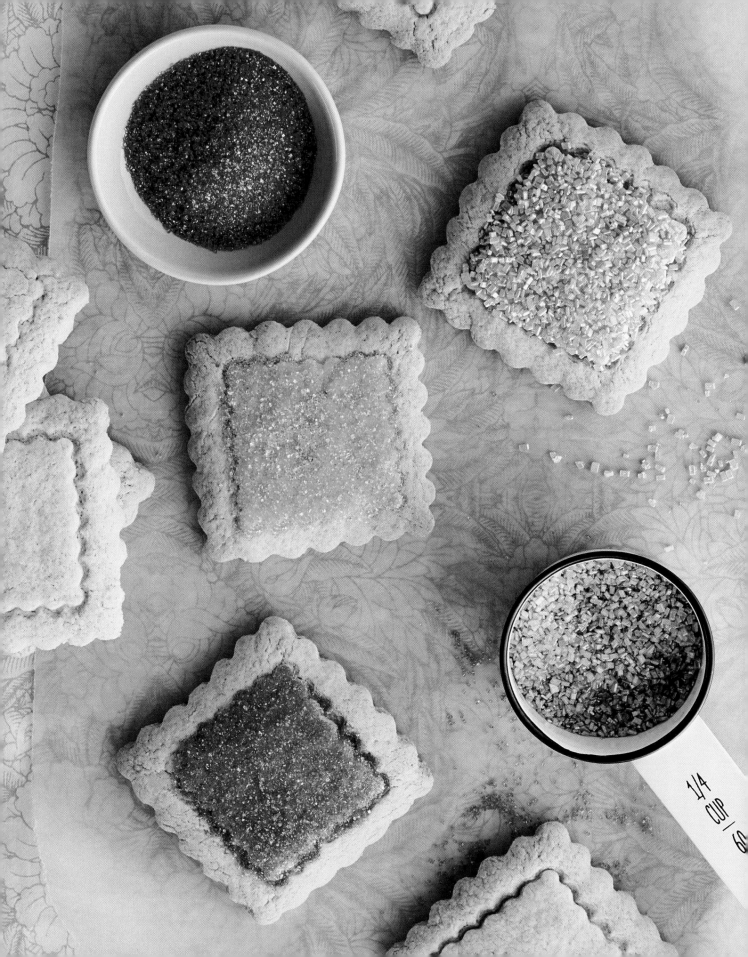

Cookies, bars and squares are a childhood treat. For many of us, one of our first treats as a toddler was likely some type of cookie. Sending a homemade cookie or treat with your family members reminds them you care and that they're important. So important, in fact, that you've made something healthy from scratch for them! Bake some "love," and send it along with your loved ones, wherever they're going. Whether it's homemade chocolate chip, raisin oatmeal, molasses, gingerbread or sugar cookies, these yummy baked goods are almost always filled with delicious sweet fruit, nuts, chocolate and other ingredients that just make you feel good. Cookies and handheld treats may also be pleasantly addictive. With the right ingredients, they can be not only tasty and gluten-free, but also nutritious. Who knew? The perfect reward.

Cookies, bars and squares make handheld treats that are easy to wrap little fingers around or satisfy big appetites. Want to eat your veggies? Try Ginger Squash Molasses Cookies (page 15) or Carrot Apricot Squares (page 27). No time to bake? Try no-bake options such as Cranberry Lemon Millet Quinoa Squares (page 36), Cranberry Almond Energy Bites (page 26) or Apricot, Walnut and Pine Nut Granola Bars (page 29). Chocolate lovers will enjoy Espresso Cookie Bars with Honey Marshmallow Meringue (page 38) and Chocolate Hazelnut Brownies (page 41). Classic favorites such as Chocolate Whoopie Pies (page 21), Oat Fig Newtons (page 18) and Chewy Raisin Oatmeal Chia Cookies (page 6) are also sure winners.

Carrot Butterscotch Cookies

A fluffy white cookie made with oat, sorghum and quinoa flours,
packed with shredded carrots and bursting with butterscotch flavor in every bite.

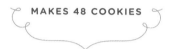

MAKES 48 COOKIES

1 cup (250 mL) finely
    ground oat flour

½ cup (125 mL) sorghum flour

½ cup (125 mL) quinoa flour

2 tsp (10 mL) baking powder

½ cup (125 mL) unsalted butter,
    softened

¼ cup (60 mL) virgin coconut oil

¾ cup (175 mL) lightly packed
    brown sugar

⅓ cup (75 mL) unsweetened
    applesauce

2 tsp (10 mL) pure vanilla extract

2 large eggs

1 cup (250 mL) raw shredded
    carrots)

¾ cup (175 mL)
    butterscotch chips

Lightly spray with cooking oil or grease two large baking sheets. Line the baking sheets with parchment paper. Preheat the oven to 350°F (180°C).

Mix together the oat, sorghum and quinoa flours and baking powder in a large bowl and set aside. In a separate medium bowl, mix the butter and coconut oil with the sugar, applesauce and vanilla. Beat in the eggs one at a time. Mix in the carrots and butterscotch chips. Add the butter mixture to the flour mixture and stir until well combined. Scoop the dough into 1 ½-inch (4 cm) balls and place them on the prepared baking sheets 2 inches (5 cm) apart.

Bake for 15 to 17 minutes, until the edges are slightly golden. Remove from the oven and allow to cool completely on the baking sheets.

PER SERVING: Energy 70 calories; Protein 1 g; Carbohydrates 8 g; Dietary Fiber 1 g; Fat 4.5 g; Sugar 4 g; Cholesterol 15 mg; Sodium 10 mg

STORAGE
Room Temperature: airtight container, 1 week
Freezer: airtight freezer container, 1 month

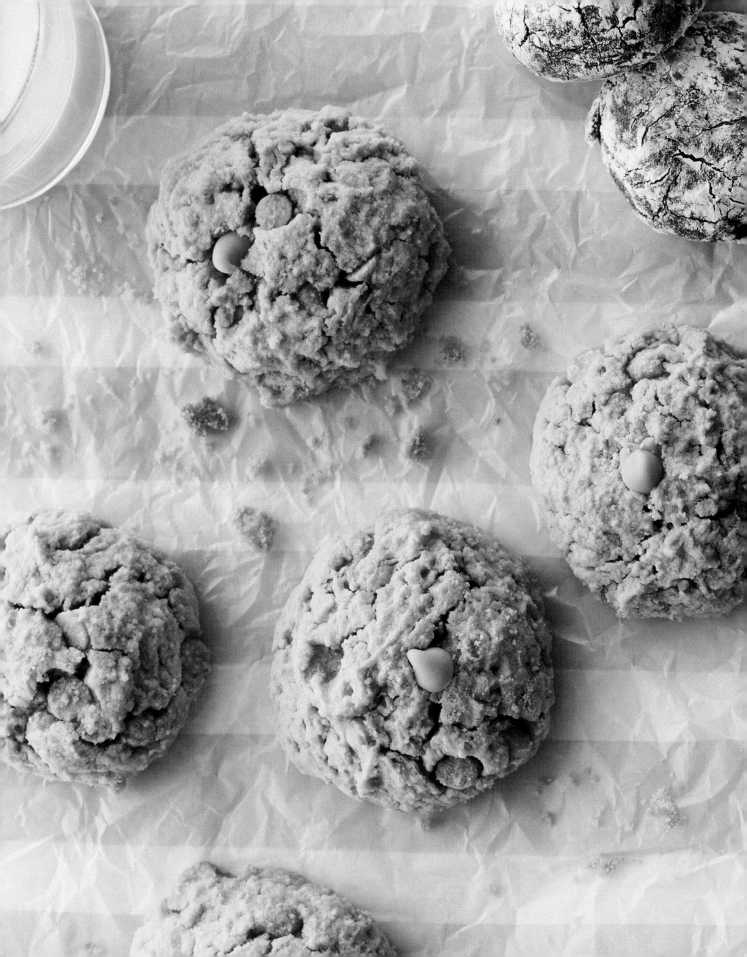

Chewy Raisin Oatmeal Chia Cookies

The dictionary definition of homemade comfort could easily be defined as freshly baked oatmeal cookies. Throw in some hazelnut flour for a gluten-free nutrition boost! These oat and chia cookies have a slight hint of cinnamon and plump raisins, and will stay fresh in the refrigerator or can be kept in the freezer and removed for quick warm-ups. Milk chocolate chips can be used in place of raisins.

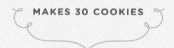

MAKES 30 COOKIES

2 Tbsp (30 mL) ground chia seeds

⅓ cup (75 mL) warm water

1 cup (250 mL) unsalted butter, softened

1 cup (250 mL) lightly packed brown sugar

½ cup (125 mL) organic cane sugar or ground Sucanat

2 large eggs

1 Tbsp (15 mL) pure vanilla extract

1 cup (250 mL) sorghum flour

½ cup (125 mL) hazelnut flour

1 tsp (5 mL) salt

1 tsp (5 mL) baking powder

½ tsp (2 mL) cinnamon

3 cups (750 mL) quick oats

1 ½ cups (375 mL) seedless raisins

Lightly spray with cooking oil or grease a large baking sheet. Line the baking sheet with parchment paper.

Stir the chia into the warm water and set aside for 10 minutes, or until thickened. Cream the butter and sugars in a large bowl. Add the chia mixture, eggs and vanilla. Stir until the ingredients are incorporated, or use a hand-mixer. Set aside. Whisk together the sorghum and hazelnut flours, salt, baking powder and cinnamon in a medium bowl. Blend half the flour mixture in with the butter mixture, then mix in the remaining flour mixture until all the dry ingredients are incorporated. Mix the oats and raisins into the dough. Cover and refrigerate for 1 hour.

Preheat the oven to 350°F (180°C).

Let the dough soften slightly, but don't let it come to room temperature. Scoop out 2 Tbsp (30 mL) of dough, roll it into a ball and flatten it into a 3-inch (8 cm) cookie. Place the cookies on the prepared baking sheet 1 inch (2.5 cm) apart.

Bake for 12 to 15 minutes, until the bottoms are golden. Do not overbake. Remove from the oven and allow the cookies to rest on the baking sheet for at least 1 minute before transferring to a rack to cool.

PER SERVING: Energy 170 calories; Protein 3 g; Carbohydrates 22 g; Dietary Fiber 2 g; Fat 7 g; Sugar 10 g; Cholesterol 30 mg; Sodium 85 mg

STORAGE

Room Temperature: airtight container or bag, 1 week

Refrigerator: airtight container or bag, 1 week

Freezer: airtight freezer bag or container, 1 month

Oat, Strawberry and Cream Cheese Thumbprint Cookies

This shortbread–like thumbprint cookie is made with oat, quinoa and sorghum flours and has a delicious cream cheese and sweet strawberry preserve center.

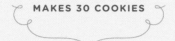

MAKES 30 COOKIES

Lightly spray with cooking oil or grease a large baking sheet. Line the baking sheet with parchment paper. Preheat the oven to 350°F (180°C).

Combine the oat, sorghum and quinoa flours and tapioca starch in a large bowl and set aside. Mix the butter and coconut oil with the sugar and vanilla in a medium bowl. Add the butter mixture to the flour mixture and stir until well combined. Roll the dough into 1 ½-inch (4 cm) balls and place them on the prepared baking sheet 1 inch (2.5 cm) apart. Press your thumb or index finger gently into the top of each cookie to make a dent. (Resist the temptation to flatten these cookies or they will spread too much when baking.) Place ¼ tsp (1 mL) of strawberry preserves then ¼ tsp (1 mL) of cream cheese in each hole.

Bake for 16 to 18 minutes, until the edges are slightly golden. Remove from the oven and allow to cool completely on the baking sheet.

⅔ cup (150 mL) oat flour

⅔ cup (150 mL) sorghum flour

⅓ cup (75 mL) quinoa flour
    (or light buckwheat flour)

⅓ cup (75 mL) tapioca starch

⅓ cup (75 mL) unsalted butter,
    softened

⅓ cup (75 mL) virgin coconut oil

½ cup (125 mL) organic
    cane sugar

1 tsp (5 mL) pure vanilla extract

2 Tbsp (30 mL) strawberry
    preserves, jam or fruit spread

2 Tbsp (30 mL) cream cheese

PER SERVING: Energy 80 calories; Protein 1 g; Carbohydrates 9 g; Dietary Fiber 1 g; Fat 5 g; Sugar 3 g; Cholesterol 5 mg; Sodium 0 mg

STORAGE

Room Temperature: airtight container, 1 week

Refrigerator: airtight container, 1 week

Freezer: airtight freezer container, 1 month

Monster Oat Chia Cookies

This is a soft, chewy cookie with colorful candy-coated milk chocolate pieces.
It's a wonderfully fun treat enhanced with more nutritional ingredients!

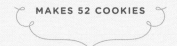

MAKES 52 COOKIES

2 Tbsp (30 mL) ground chia seeds

½ cup (125 mL) boiling water

½ cup (125 mL) unsalted butter, softened

½ cup (125 mL) lightly packed brown sugar

½ cup (125 mL) organic cane sugar

2 large eggs

1 Tbsp (15 mL) pure vanilla extract

¾ cup (175 mL) old-fashioned rolled oats

1 cup (250 mL) oat flour

½ cup (125 mL) millet flour

½ cup (125 mL) coconut flour

½ tsp (2 mL) baking soda

1 tsp (5 mL) cinnamon

½ tsp (2 mL) salt

1 ¼ cups (310 mL) candy-coated milk chocolate pieces

Grease or spray with cooking oil a large baking sheet and line with parchment paper. Preheat the oven to 375°F (190°C).

Add the chia to the boiling water in a small bowl. Gently stir with a fork to ensure the ground seeds are evenly distributed. Set aside to thicken, about 10 minutes.

Cream the butter and sugars in a large bowl. Add the chia mixture, eggs and vanilla and stir until the mixture has a smooth consistency.

In a separate bowl, mix the oats with the oat, millet and coconut flours, baking soda, cinnamon and salt. Add the butter mixture to the flour mixture and mix well to combine. Stir in the candy-coated chocolate pieces. Drop by oversized tablespoons (or use a 1 ½-inch/4 cm scoop) on the baking sheet 2 inches (5 cm) apart. Flatten them slightly with the palm of your hand.

Bake for 10 to 12 minutes, until the edges are slightly golden brown. Allow the cookies to set for 5 minutes on the baking sheet before transferring them to a rack to cool completely.

PER SERVING: Energy 80 calories; Protein 1 g; Carbohydrates 10 g; Dietary Fiber 1 g; Fat 3 g; Sugar 7 g; Cholesterol 15 mg; Sodium 45 mg

STORAGE

Room Temperature: airtight container, 1 week

Refrigerator: airtight container, 10 days

Freezer: airtight freezer bag or container, 1 month

Chocolate Whirl Cookies

These clever cookies are half double chocolate, half regular chocolate chip. Not only do they look great and taste chocolaty, they are soft and chewy and made with sorghum, oat and quinoa flours!

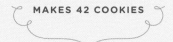

MAKES 42 COOKIES

Grease or spray with cooking oil a large baking sheet. Line the baking sheet with parchment paper. Preheat the oven to 350°F (180°C).

Combine the sorghum, oat and quinoa flours, baking soda and salt in a large bowl and set aside. In a separate medium bowl, cream the butter and sugar. Add the eggs, applesauce, maple syrup and vanilla. Mix well until the mixture has a smooth consistency.

Add the butter mixture to the flour mixture and mix well. Divide the batter evenly in two, placing each half in a separate bowl. Add the chocolate chips to one bowl. Add the cocoa powder and mix in the white chocolate chips in the other bowl. Using a 1 ½-inch (4 cm) scoop, fill half the scoop with the regular chocolate chip dough and the other half with the double chocolate chip dough. Place the dough balls on the prepared baking sheet 2 inches (5 cm) apart.

Bake for 8 to 10 minutes, until the cookies just start to turn golden on the edges. Do not overbake. Allow the cookies to set for 10 minutes on the baking sheet before moving to a rack to cool completely.

PER SERVING: Energy 80 calories; Protein 1 g; Carbohydrates 9 g; Dietary Fiber 1 g; Fat 5 g; Sugar 5 g; Cholesterol 20 mg; Sodium 65 mg

⅔ cup (150 mL) sorghum flour

⅔ cup (150 mL) oat flour

⅔ cup (150 mL) quinoa flour

1 tsp (5 mL) baking soda

½ tsp (2 mL) salt

¾ cup (175 mL) unsalted butter, softened

½ cup (125 mL) lightly packed brown sugar

2 large eggs

¼ cup (60 mL) unsweetened applesauce

2 Tbsp (30 mL) pure maple syrup

2 tsp (10 mL) pure vanilla extract

½ cup (125 mL) semisweet chocolate chips

2 Tbsp (30 mL) unsweetened cocoa powder

½ cup (125 mL) white chocolate chips

STORAGE

Refrigerator: **airtight container or bag, 10 days**

Freezer: **airtight freezer bag or container, 1 month**

BAKING TIP

· Maximize your antioxidants by using regular unsweetened cocoa powder and avoiding Dutch process cocoa, where many of the useful antioxidants have been destroyed.

· Be unrefined! We also use organic whole brown muscovado sugar (fair trade) instead of regular brown sugar.

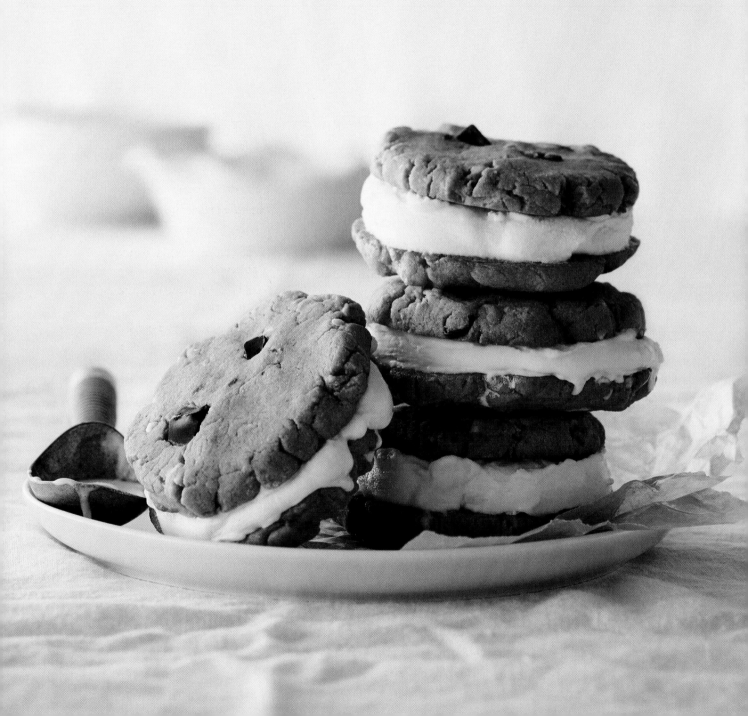

Peanut Butter
Chocolate Chunk Cookies

Looking for cookies that still taste fresh-baked and chewy days after baking? Sorghum and psyllium help make these delicious cookies nutritious. Your friends will leave you only the crumbs. We love these cookies in ice cream sandwiches.

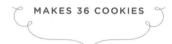

MAKES 36 COOKIES

Line a large baking sheet with parchment paper. Preheat the oven to 350°F (180°C).

Whisk together the sorghum and quinoa flours, tapioca starch, psyllium, baking powder and salt in a medium bowl. Set aside.

In a separate large bowl, beat the butter with the brown sugar until well combined. Beat in the peanut butter, then one egg at a time, followed by the vanilla. Stir in the flour mixture gradually until fully incorporated (the dough may appear oily, but gluten-free flours combined with natural peanut butter make it look that way). Work in the chocolate chunks and peanut pieces until evenly distributed.

Using 2 Tbsp (30 mL) of dough per cookie, roll the dough into balls. Flatten to ½ inch (1 cm) thick and reform into a circle if necessary. Place the cookies on the prepared baking sheet 1 inch (2.5 cm) apart.

Bake for 8 for 9 minutes, until the bottoms are golden. Allow to cool on the baking sheet for 1 minute. Transfer to a wire rack to cool completely.

PER SERVING: Energy 190 calories; Protein 2 g; Carbohydrates 17 g; Dietary Fiber 1 g; Fat 9 g; Sugar 7 g; Cholesterol 15 mg; Sodium 55 mg

1 cup (250 mL) sorghum flour

½ cup (125 mL) quinoa flour

½ cup (125 mL) tapioca starch

2 tsp (10 mL) psyllium husks

1 tsp (5 mL) baking powder

½ tsp (2 mL) salt

½ cup (125 mL) unsalted butter, softened

1 cup (250 mL) lightly packed brown sugar

1 cup (250 mL) natural peanut butter (smooth or crunchy), stirred well

2 large eggs

1 Tbsp (15 mL) pure vanilla extract

⅔ cup (150 mL) semisweet chocolate chunks

½ cup (125 mL) chopped, unsalted peanuts

STORAGE

Room Temperature: airtight container or bag, 2 weeks

Refrigerator: airtight container or bag, 2 weeks

Freezer: airtight freezer bag or container, 1 month

Mocha Crinkle Cookies

This soft mocha cookie rolled in powdered (icing) sugar is a real treat with the nutritional enhancement of sorghum flour. The more chilled the dough, the bigger the crinkles and cracks will be. Make your cookies as crinkly as you want! Make your own powdered sugar if you like (see recipe on facing page).

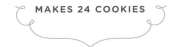

MAKES 24 COOKIES

¾ cup (175 mL) sorghum flour

½ cup (125 mL) tapioca starch

½ cup (125 mL) unsweetened cocoa powder

2 tsp (10 mL) psyllium husks

2 tsp (10 mL) instant coffee powder

¾ tsp (3 mL) baking powder

¼ tsp (1 mL) salt

⅔ cup (150 mL) lightly packed brown sugar

½ cup (125 mL) grapeseed oil

1 large egg

1 large egg white

2 tsp (10 mL) pure vanilla extract

¼ cup (60 mL) powdered (icing) sugar, in a shallow bowl

Line a large baking sheet with parchment paper. Preheat the oven to 350°F (180°C).

Whisk together the sorghum flour, tapioca starch, cocoa, psyllium, coffee powder, baking powder and salt in a medium bowl. Set aside.

In a separate large bowl, beat the brown sugar with the oil, egg, egg white and vanilla. Gradually add the flour mixture to the egg mixture until well combined. Cover the dough and refrigerate for 2 hours. The dough must be completely chilled when you use it for the cookies to crack properly. Roll the dough into 1 ¼-inch (3 cm) balls and then roll them in the powdered sugar. Place the cookies on the prepared baking sheet 1 ½ inches (4 cm) apart.

Bake for 9 to 10 minutes, until the tops have cracked. Remove from the oven and allow to cool on the baking sheet for 1 minute. Transfer to a rack to cool completely.

PER SERVING: Energy 100 calories; Protein 1 g; Carbohydrates 13 g; Dietary Fiber 2 g; Fat 5 g; Sugar 5 g; Cholesterol 10 mg; Sodium 30 mg

BAKING TIP
The colder the dough is when baked the larger the cracks, but don't use frozen dough.

STORAGE
Room Temperature: slightly open container or bag, 5 days

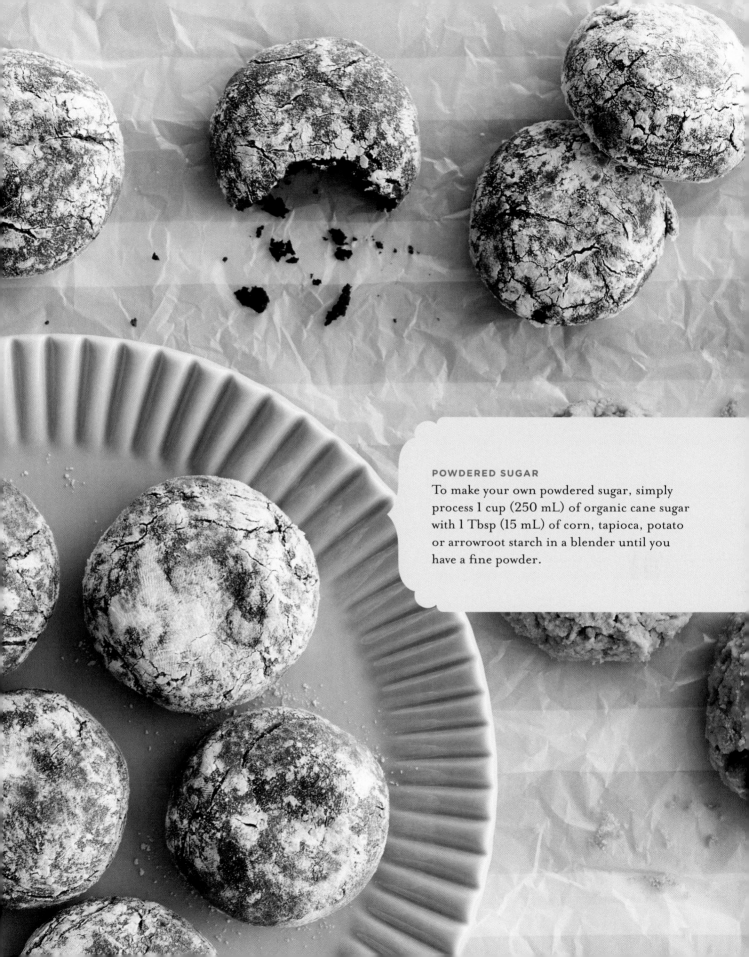

POWDERED SUGAR
To make your own powdered sugar, simply process 1 cup (250 mL) of organic cane sugar with 1 Tbsp (15 mL) of corn, tapioca, potato or arrowroot starch in a blender until you have a fine powder.

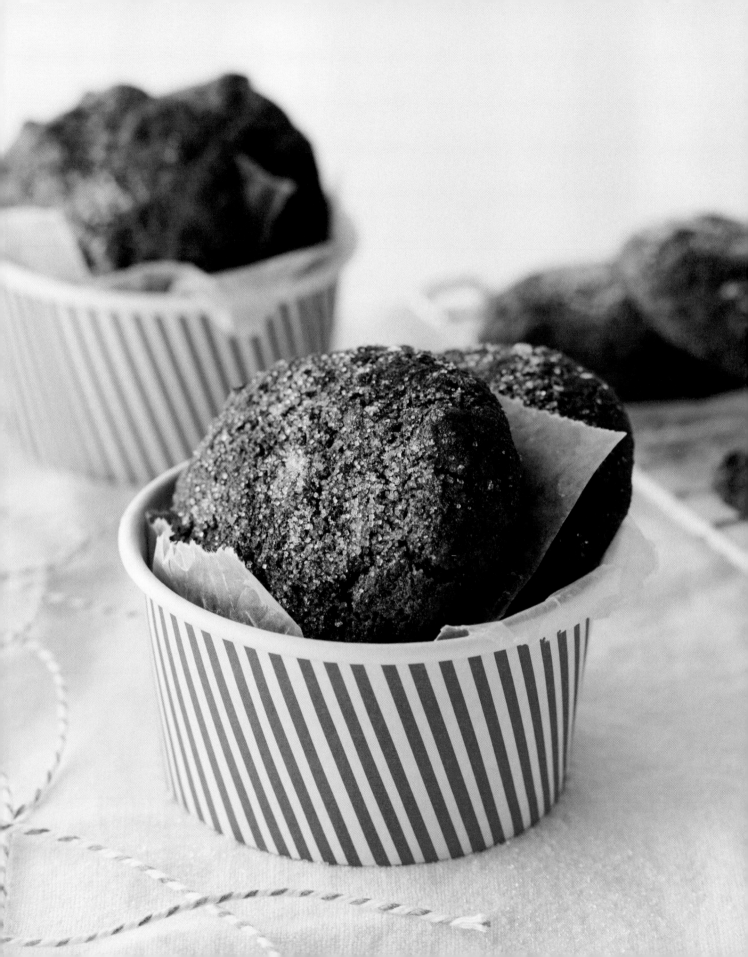

Ginger Squash Molasses Cookies

These are large, soft molasses cookies enhanced with the nutrition of teff, sorghum and butternut squash!

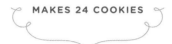

MAKES 24 COOKIES

Line a large baking sheet with parchment paper. Preheat the oven to 350°F (180°C).

Whisk together the sorghum and teff flours, baking soda, cinnamon, ginger, xanthan gum, cloves and salt in a medium bowl and set aside. In a separate large bowl, mix together the brown sugar, squash, oil, eggs and molasses until smooth. Slowly add the flour mixture to the squash mixture, stirring until thoroughly combined.

Using a ¼ cup (60 mL) scoop or measuring cup, drop the cookie dough onto the prepared baking sheet 1 ½ inches (4 cm) apart. Sprinkle the tops with a pinch of cane sugar.

Bake for 12 to 15 minutes, or until a toothpick inserted in the center comes out clean. Allow the cookies to sit for 2 minutes on the sheet before moving them to a rack to cool completely.

PER SERVING: Energy 140 calories; Protein 2 g; Carbohydrates 21 g; Dietary Fiber 2 g; Fat 6 g; Sugar 10 g; Cholesterol 15 mg; Sodium 190 mg

1 ½ cups (375 mL) sorghum flour

1 cup (250 mL) teff flour

4 tsp (20 mL) baking soda

4 tsp (20 mL) cinnamon

2 tsp (10 mL) ground ginger

1 ½ tsp (7 mL) xanthan gum

1 tsp (5 mL) ground cloves

½ tsp (2 mL) salt

1 cup (250 mL) lightly packed
   brown sugar

1 cup (250 mL) cooked butternut
   squash or pure pumpkin puree

½ cup (125 mL) grapeseed oil

2 large eggs

¼ cup (60 mL) molasses

3 Tbsp (45 mL) organic
   cane sugar

STORAGE
Room Temperature: airtight container, 1 week
Refrigerator: airtight container, 1 week
Freezer: airtight freezer bag or container, 1 month

Triple Chocolate Coconut Chia Cookies

A blend of sorghum, millet and coconut flours is the base for these cookies, loaded with milk and white chocolate. Coconut oil with chia makes them moist, chewy, super soft — and extra tasty.

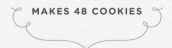

MAKES 48 COOKIES

1 Tbsp (15 mL) ground chia seeds

¼ cup (60 mL) boiling water

¾ cup (175 mL) virgin coconut oil

1 ¼ cups (310 mL) lightly packed brown sugar

4 large eggs

1 tsp (5 mL) pure vanilla extract

¾ cup (175 mL) sorghum flour

¾ cup (175 mL) millet flour

½ cup (125 mL) coconut flour

½ cup (125 mL) tapioca starch

⅔ cup (150 mL) unsweetened cocoa powder

2 tsp (10 mL) baking soda

½ tsp (2 mL) salt

1 ½ cups (375 mL) white chocolate chips

½ cup (125 mL) semisweet or milk chocolate chips

Grease a large baking sheet or line it with parchment paper. Preheat the oven to 375°F (190°C).

Add the chia to the boiling water in a small bowl. Gently stir with a fork to ensure the ground seeds are evenly distributed. Set aside to thicken, about 10 minutes.

Cream the coconut oil with the brown sugar in a large bowl. Add the chia mixture, eggs and vanilla. Mix well until the mixture has a smooth consistency. Set aside.

In a separate large bowl, mix together the sorghum, millet and coconut flours, tapioca starch, cocoa, baking soda and salt. Add the butter mixture to the flour mixture and mix well to combine. Stir in all the chocolate chips. Roll the dough into 1 ¼-inch (3 cm) balls and place them on the prepared baking sheet 2 inches (5 cm) apart. Flatten each ball slightly with the palm of your hand.

Bake for 8 to 10 minutes, until puffed and set. Allow the cookies to set for 5 minutes on the baking sheet before transferring to a rack to cool completely.

PER SERVING: Energy 120 calories; Protein 2 g; Carbohydrates 13 g; Dietary Fiber 1 g; Fat 6 g; Sugar 8 g; Cholesterol 15 mg; Sodium 80 mg

STORAGE

Room Temperature: airtight container or bag, 1 week

Freezer: airtight freezer bag or container, 1 month

Salted Caramel Pecan Shortbread Bites

A buttery shortbread made with sorghum and millet flours, and topped with caramel and coarse salt for a luxurious, pop-straight-in-your-mouth bite-sized cookie.

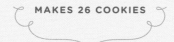

MAKES 26 COOKIES

For the caramel, bring the brown sugar, cream and 2 Tbsp (30 mL) butter to a boil in a medium saucepan. Turn down the heat to a simmer and continue to cook for 5 minutes, stirring frequently. Remove from the heat and set aside to cool.

Lightly spray with cooking oil or grease a large baking sheet. Line the baking sheet with parchment paper. Preheat the oven to 350°F (180°C).

Combine the sorghum and millet flours, tapioca starch, salt, butter, sugar and vanilla with the pecans in a large bowl. Roll the dough into 1 ½-inch (4 cm) balls and place them on the prepared baking sheet 1 inch (2.5 cm) apart. Press your thumb gently into the top of each cookie. Drop ¼–½ tsp (1–2 mL) of caramel sauce into each dent and sprinkle with salt.

Bake for 16 to 18 minutes, until the edges are slightly golden. Remove from the oven and allow to cool completely on the baking sheet.

PER SERVING: Energy 120 calories; Protein 1 g; Carbohydrates 12 g; Dietary Fiber 1 g; Fat 7 g; Sugar 6 g; Cholesterol 15 mg; Sodium 290 mg

CARAMEL

⅓ cup (75 mL) lightly packed brown sugar

¼ cup (60 mL) 5% cream

2 Tbsp (30 mL) unsalted butter

PECAN SHORTBREAD BITES

¾ cup (175 mL) sorghum flour

½ cup (125 mL) millet flour

½ cup (125 mL) tapioca starch

¼ tsp (1 mL) salt

¼ cup (60 mL) unsalted butter, softened

½ cup (125 mL) organic cane sugar

2 tsp (10 mL) pure vanilla extract

¼ cup (60 mL) finely chopped pecans

2 Tbsp (30 mL) coarse salt

BAKING TIP
Short on time? Make the caramel the day before and refrigerate it overnight. You can use it straight from the refrigerator.

STORAGE
Room Temperature: airtight container or bag, 1 week
Freezer: airtight freezer bag or container, 1 month

Oat Fig Newtons

*Full of luscious pureed figs, this all-time favorite is
gluten-free with the help of wholesome oat and sorghum flours.*

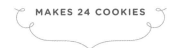

MAKES 24 COOKIES

DOUGH

½ cup (125 mL) oat flour

½ cup (125 mL) sorghum flour

½ cup (125 mL) tapioca starch

¼ cup (60 mL) unsalted butter,
    softened

⅓ cup (75 mL) organic
    cane sugar

1 large egg

2 tsp (10 mL) pure vanilla extract

FILLING

2 cups (500 mL) dried figs

⅓ cup (75 mL) fresh orange juice

½ tsp (2 mL) fresh orange zest

1 Tbsp (15 mL) liquid honey

Lightly spray or grease a large baking sheet. Line the baking sheet
with parchment paper.

For the dough, whisk together the oat and sorghum flours and
tapioca starch. Set aside. Cream the butter with the sugar, egg
and vanilla in a medium bowl. Add the butter mixture to the flour
mixture, stirring until a dough forms. Roll the dough into a ball,
wrap in plastic wrap and place in the refrigerator for 30 minutes.

For the filling, place the figs, orange juice and zest and honey
with 1 cup (250 mL) of water in a medium saucepan over medium
heat. Bring to a boil and then reduce to a simmer. Cook for 5 to
8 minutes, until most of the seeds have separated from the skins.
Set the mixture aside to cool. Using a food processor or immersion
blender, puree the mixture until it becomes a smooth jam or paste.
Set aside.

Preheat the oven to 350°F (180°C).

Take the dough out of the refrigerator and place it on a floured
piece of parchment or wax paper (this helps to bend and shape
dough away from a hard surface such as a countertop). Roll the
dough into a 12-inch (30 cm) square. Cut the square of dough
into three 4-inch (10 cm) wide strips. Spread fig puree along the
middle of each length of dough. Roll from the long edge in to
create a log, pinching to seal. Trim the ends and cut each log into
eight 1 ½-inch (4 cm) individual cookies. Place the cookies on the
prepared baking sheet ½ inch (1 cm) apart.

Bake for 16 to 18 minutes, until the edges are lightly golden.
Allow to cool completely on the baking sheet.

PER SERVING: Energy 90 calories; Protein 1 g; Carbohydrates 17 g;
Dietary Fiber 2 g; Fat 2.5 g; Sugar 10 g; Cholesterol 15 mg; Sodium 0 mg

STORAGE

Refrigerator: airtight container, 1 week

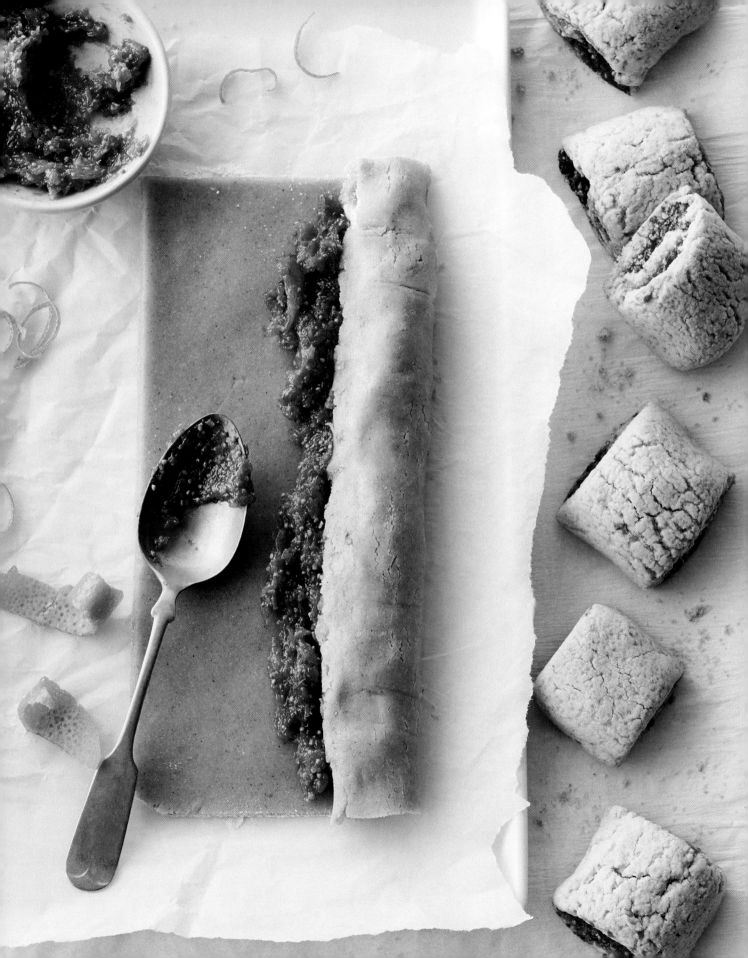

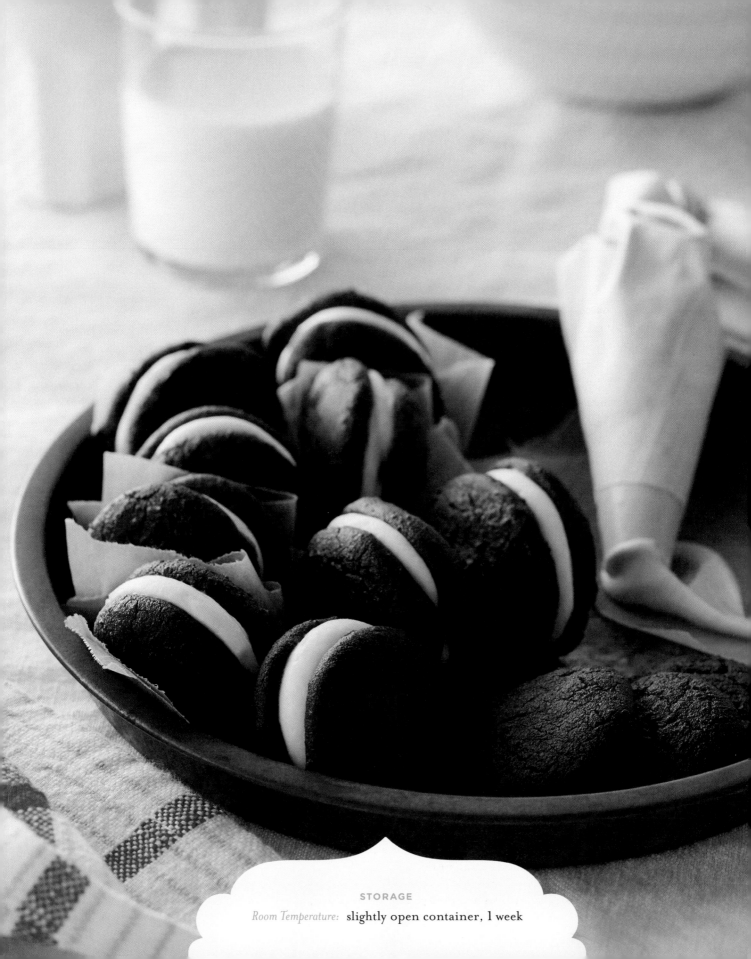

Chocolate Whoopie Pies

Many variations of whoopie pies have been a tradition in North America for years, with all kinds of names. One thing we can agree on is that these deliciously soft chocolate cookies are fabulous for any family occasion, especially picnics.

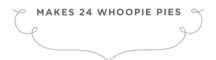

MAKES 24 WHOOPIE PIES

For the cookies, place the quinoa in a medium saucepan with 1 cup (250 mL) of water and bring to a boil. Turn down the heat to a simmer, cover and cook for 15 minutes. Remove from the heat and let sit, covered, for an additional 15 minutes. The quinoa seeds will be very fluffy when cooked.

Line a large baking sheet with parchment paper. Preheat the oven to 350°F (180°C).

Whisk together the sorghum and rice flours, cocoa, psyllium, baking soda and salt in a large bowl until combined. Set aside.

Place the fluffy cooked quinoa in a blender with the milk, eggs and vanilla. Blend for a few moments then add the melted butter. Continue to blend until the mixture is completely smooth with no whole quinoa remaining in the batter. Blend in the brown sugar until thoroughly incorporated. Add the pureed batter to the flour mixture. Mix until fully combined and there is a smooth dough.

Using a tablespoon, scoop the dough onto the prepared baking sheet, leaving about 1 ½ inches (4 cm) between each cookie.

Bake for 15 for 17 minutes, until the bottoms are golden. Allow the cookies to cool on the sheet for a few minutes, until they can easily be transferred to a rack to cool completely.

For the filling, whip the egg white and cream of tartar on high speed in a stand mixer until soft peaks form. Set aside.

Place the sugar and honey in a saucepan with 1 Tbsp (15 mL) of water and bring to a simmer. Simmer for about 1 ½ minutes while whisking, until the sugar has completely dissolved. Restart the stand mixer and pour the hot syrup 1 Tbsp (15 mL) at a time into the whipped egg whites with the machine running. Do this until all the syrup is gone. Whip for another 7 minutes, until this marshmallow cream has become glossy with stiff peaks. Use 1 ½ tsp (7 mL) of filling to sandwich together two cookies. Store the cookies with layers separated by parchment or wax paper.

COOKIES

½ cup (125 mL) quinoa seeds

1 cup (250 mL) sorghum flour

½ cup (125 mL) brown rice
   or white rice flour

½ cup (125 mL) unsweetened
   cocoa powder

2 tsp (10 mL) psyllium husks

1 tsp (5 mL) baking soda

½ tsp (2 mL) salt

1 cup (250 mL) 1% milk
   or water

2 large eggs

2 tsp (10 mL) pure vanilla extract

⅔ cup (150 mL) unsalted butter,
   melted

1 cup (250 mL) lightly packed
   brown sugar

FILLING

1 large egg white

⅛ tsp (0.5 mL) cream of tartar

½ cup (125 mL) organic
   cane sugar

1 Tbsp (15 mL) honey

PER SERVING: Energy 180 calories; Protein 3 g; Carbohydrates 25 g; Dietary Fiber 2 g; Fat 9 g; Sugar 13 g; Cholesterol 35 mg; Sodium 114 mg

Mint Matcha Morsels

These mini morsels of chocolaty goodness are perfect for the moments when you need something small and quick to eat on the run. Dark chocolate, green matcha tea, coconut, oats and chia, slightly sweetened with honey, make a perfect snack when you need a chocolate fix. Stow them in your purse or yoga bag for emergencies.

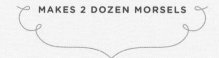

MAKES 2 DOZEN MORSELS

1 egg white

¼ tsp (1 mL) peppermint extract

½ cup (125 mL) quality semisweet chocolate pieces or chips

1 Tbsp (15 mL) liquid honey

½ cup (125 mL) unsweetened flaked coconut

½ cup (125 mL) quick oats or quinoa flakes

2 Tbsp (30 mL) chia seeds

½ tsp (2 mL) green matcha tea powder

Line a large baking sheet with parchment paper. Preheat the oven to 300°F (150°C).

Whisk together the egg white and peppermint extract and set aside.

Melt the chocolate and honey in a double boiler. Remove from the heat and let cool slightly. Gradually add the egg white mixture, whisking all the time. Stir in the coconut, oats, chia and matcha, being sure to coat everything completely. Use a tablespoon to scoop the mixture onto the prepared baking sheet, leaving 1 inch (2.5 cm) of space between each scoop. Reshape into balls if necessary.

Bake for 15 minutes.

Allow the morsels to cool for at least 2 minutes before removing them from the sheet.

PER SERVING: Energy 45 calories; Protein 1 g; Carbohydrates 6 g; Dietary Fiber 1 g; Fat 2.5 g; Sugar 3 g; Cholesterol 0 mg; Sodium 25 mg

STORAGE

Room Temperature: airtight container, 1 month

Refrigerator: airtight container, 1 month

Double Chocolate Sorghum and Teff Biscotti

*Ready to dip. A sorghum and teff flour blend makes these airy
and crunchy biscotti gluten-free and as tasty as ever.*

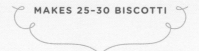

MAKES 25-30 BISCOTTI

Lightly spray with cooking oil or grease a large baking sheet.
Line the baking sheet with parchment paper. Preheat the oven
to 350°F (180°C).

Mix together the sorghum and teff flours, tapioca starch, cocoa,
baking powder, baking soda and salt in a large bowl. Add the
chocolate chips. Set aside.

In a separate medium bowl, beat the butter with the sugar. Add
the eggs and vanilla and blend well. Add the butter mixture to
the flour mixture and stir until well combined. Divide the dough
in half and roll it into long logs, the same length as the prepared
baking sheet. With slightly damp hands, gently pat the dough
to flatten each log until it is ¾ inch (2 cm) thick and 10 inches
(25 cm) long.

Bake for 20 minutes.

Remove from the oven and let sit until cool enough to touch.
Slice each log into 1-inch (2.5 cm) pieces. Place the slices on the
same baking sheet and bake for an additional 6 minutes on each
side. Remove from the oven and allow to cool slightly on the
baking sheet before moving to a wire rack to cool completely
and harden.

PER SERVING: Energy 100 calories; Protein 2 g; Carbohydrates 14 g;
Dietary Fiber 1 g; Fat 4 g; Sugar 6 g; Cholesterol 30 mg; Sodium 60 mg

¾ cup (175 mL) sorghum flour

½ cup (125 mL) teff flour

½ cup (125 mL) tapioca starch

¼ cup (60 mL) unsweetened
cocoa powder

½ tsp (2 mL) baking powder

½ tsp (2 mL) baking soda

¼ tsp (1 mL) salt

½ cup (125 mL) white mini
chocolate chips

¼ cup (60 mL) unsalted butter,
softened

½ cup (125 mL) organic
cane sugar

3 large eggs, beaten

2 tsp (10 mL) pure vanilla extract

STORAGE

Room Temperature: airtight container or bag, 1 week

Freezer: airtight freezer bag or container, 1 month

Citrus Sorghum and Oat Biscotti

Lemon and lime combine with fresh ginger to make these biscotti stand out from the average biscotti. Extra lovely with a drizzle of white chocolate.

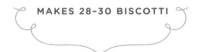

MAKES 28-30 BISCOTTI

1 cup (250 mL) sorghum flour

¾ cup (175 mL) oat flour

½ cup (125 mL) tapioca starch

½ tsp (2 mL) baking powder

½ tsp (2 mL) baking soda

¼ tsp (1 mL) salt

1 Tbsp (15 mL) grated lemon zest

¼ cup (60 mL) unsalted butter, softened

½ cup (125 mL) organic cane sugar

3 large eggs, beaten

2 tsp (10 mL) fresh lime juice

1 tsp (5 mL) grated fresh ginger

½ cup (125 mL) white mini chocolate chips

Lightly spray with cooking oil or grease a large baking sheet. Line the baking sheet with parchment paper. Preheat the oven to 350°F (180°C).

Combine the sorghum and oat flours, tapioca starch, baking powder, baking soda, salt and lemon zest in a large bowl. Set aside.

In a separate medium bowl, beat the butter with the sugar. Add the eggs, lime juice and ginger and blend well. Add the butter mixture to the flour mixture and stir until well combined. Divide the dough in half and spread it into long logs, the same length as the prepared baking sheet. With slightly damp hands, gently pat to reshape and flatten each log until it is ¾ inch (2 cm) thick and 10 inches (25 cm) long.

Bake for 20 minutes.

Remove from the oven and let sit until cool enough to touch. Slice each log horizontally into 1-inch (2.5 cm) pieces. Place the slices back on the same baking sheet and bake for an additional 6 minutes on each side. Remove from the oven and allow to cool.

Melt the white chocolate chips on low heat in a double boiler. Using a small spoon or ladle, drizzle the chocolate over the biscotti. Move to a wire rack to cool completely and harden.

PER SERVING: Energy 80 calories; Protein 2 g; Carbohydrates 12 g; Dietary Fiber 1 g; Fat 3 g; Sugar 5 g; Cholesterol 25 mg; Sodium 50 mg

BAKING TIP
Short on time? Add white mini chocolate chips to the biscotti dough instead of making the chocolate drizzle.

STORAGE

Room Temperature: airtight container or bag, 1 week

Freezer: airtight freezer bag or container, 1 month

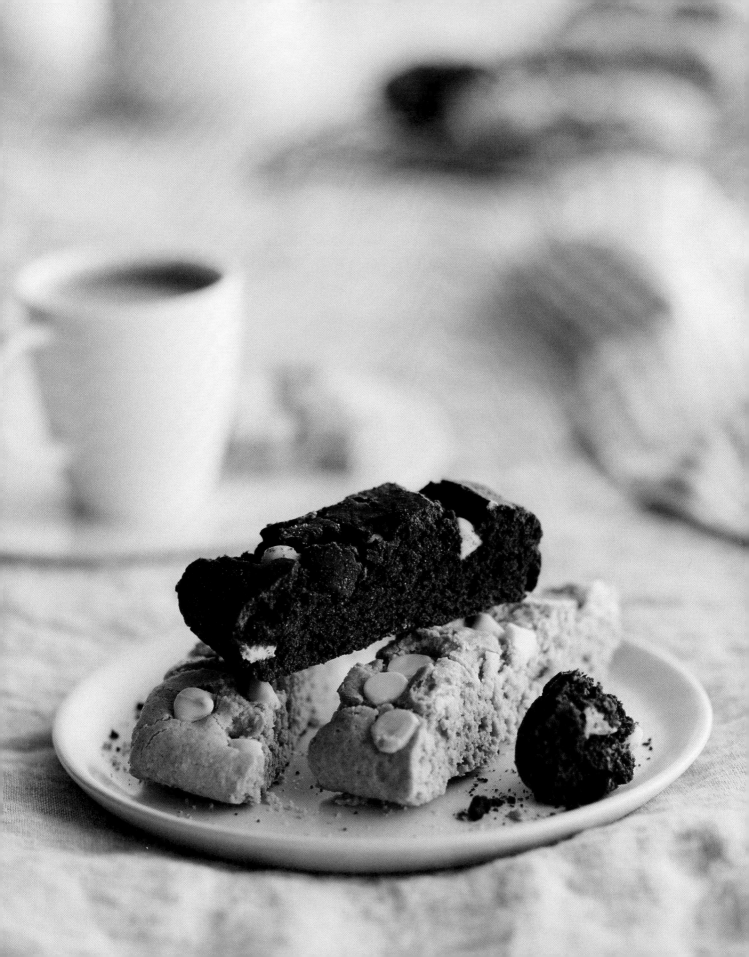

Cranberry Almond Energy Bites

On hectic days, nutrition is even more important than usual. Quinoa, oats and chia with cranberries, coconut and almonds make these delicious bites of energy. Easy to prepare and take along, these no–bake morsels will be there to snack on whenever you need them.

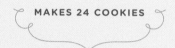

MAKES 24 COOKIES

²/₃ cup (150 mL) large-flake or quick oats

²/₃ cup (150 mL) unsweetened medium-shredded coconut

½ cup (125 mL) quinoa or amaranth flakes

½ cup (125 mL) sweetened dried cranberries, coarsely chopped

¼ cup (60 mL) chia seeds

²/₃ cup (150 mL) unsalted almond or peanut butter (crunchy or smooth)

⅓ cup (75 mL) liquid honey

2 tsp (10 mL) pure vanilla extract

Mix together the oats, coconut, quinoa flakes, cranberries and chia in a large bowl. Add the almond butter, honey and vanilla and mix well to combine. Roll the mixture into tablespoon-sized balls. And they're ready to eat.

PER SERVING: Energy 90 calories; Protein 3 g; Carbohydrates 10 g; Dietary Fiber 2 g; Fat 6 g; Sugar 4 g; Cholesterol 0 mg; Sodium 25 mg

STORAGE

Room Temperature: airtight container or bag, 2 weeks

Refrigerator: airtight container or bag, 2 weeks

Carrot Apricot Squares

These tasty squares are made with carrots, white chocolate and chewy, sweet apricots, and have a dense, moist, brownie-like texture.

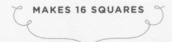

MAKES 16 SQUARES

Lightly grease an 8-inch (2 L) square baking pan. Line the bottom with parchment paper. Preheat the oven to 350°F (180°C).

Whisk together the sorghum and quinoa flours, cinnamon, ginger and salt in a medium bowl and set aside. Using a handheld mixer, beat the carrots with the eggs, sugar, orange juice and maple syrup in a separate medium bowl. Set aside.

Melt the chocolate and butter in a medium saucepan or double boiler over low heat. When the chocolate is almost completely melted, remove it from the heat and mix it into the carrot mixture. Add the carrot mixture to the flour mixture and blend well. Stir in the apricots, then pour the mixture into the prepared pan.

Bake for 30 to 35 minutes, until a toothpick inserted in the center comes out with only a few crumbs. Allow to cool completely in the pan before cutting into squares. Serve cold.

PER SERVING: Energy 130 calories; Protein 2 g; Carbohydrates 19 g; Dietary Fiber 2 g; Fat 6 g; Sugar 12 g; Cholesterol 30 mg; Sodium 45 mg

½ cup (125 mL) sorghum flour

½ cup (125 mL) quinoa flour

1 tsp (5 mL) cinnamon

½ tsp (2 mL) ground ginger

½ tsp (2 mL) salt

1 ½ cups (375 mL) cooked, pureed carrots

2 large eggs

½ cup (125 mL) lightly packed brown sugar

2 Tbsp (30 mL) fresh orange or lemon juice

1 Tbsp (15 mL) pure maple syrup

½ cup (125 mL) white chocolate chips or 4 oz (115 g) white baking chocolate

¼ cup (60 mL) unsalted butter

¾ cup (175 mL) chopped dried apricots

STORAGE

Room Temperature: airtight container, 1 week

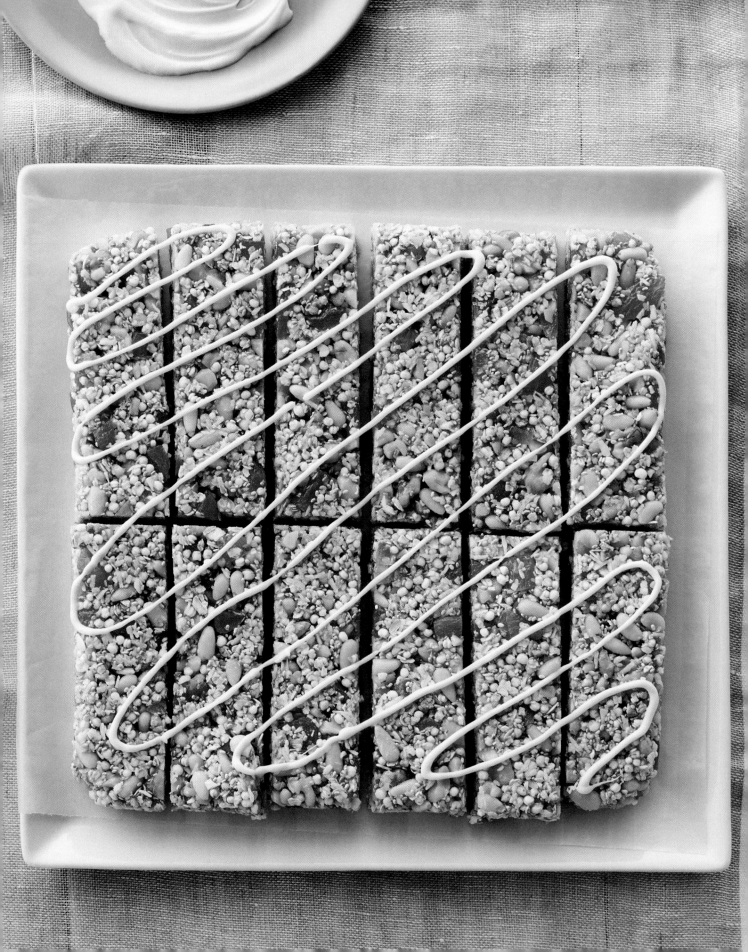

Apricot, Walnut and Pine Nut Granola Bars

Take store-bought granola bars off your grocery list! Make them easily yourself and know the nutritional benefits of snacking on them. Apricots, walnuts and pine nuts are a tasty combination and create a pleasing texture.

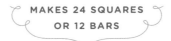

MAKES 24 SQUARES OR 12 BARS

Lightly grease a 9-inch (2.5 L) square baking dish or pan. Line the bottom and sides with one piece of parchment, big enough so that it can fold over itself to completely cover the top of the pan, and grease the parchment or lightly spray with cooking oil.

Place the dried apricots, walnuts, pine nuts, puffs, oats, coconut and chia in a large bowl and set aside.

Bring the honey to a simmer in a small saucepan for 1 minute. Remove from the heat and stir in the vanilla. Pour over the puff mixture and stir until completely covered.

Press the mixture firmly and evenly into the pan, folding in the side pieces of parchment to cover the mixture and keep your hands clean. Melt the chocolate chips in a double boiler or microwave oven (15-second intervals with stirring in between) until smooth. Place the chocolate in a small resealable plastic bag, then cut ¼ inch (1 cm) from one corner and pipe chocolate overtop the granola mix.

Cover with plastic wrap and place in the refrigerator to set for at least 1 hour. Cut into 12 bars or 24 squares.

1 cup (250 mL) finely chopped dried apricots

¾ cup (175 mL) coarsely chopped walnuts

¾ cup (175 mL) pine nuts

¾ cup (175 mL) quinoa or millet puffs

¾ cup (175 mL) quick oats

½ cup (125 mL) unsweetened finely grated coconut

¼ cup (60 mL) chia seeds

½ cup (125 mL) liquid honey

1 tsp (5 mL) pure vanilla extract

½ cup (125 mL) white chocolate chips

PER SERVING (squares): Energy 140 calories; Protein 2 g; Carbohydrates 16 g; Dietary Fiber 2 g; Fat 8 g; Sugar 11 g; Cholesterol 0 mg; Sodium 10 mg

STORAGE

Room Temperature: **slightly open container, 1 week**

Apple Raisin Oat Squares

Baked apples and raisins sandwiched between two layers of buttery oats along with ancient grain brethren chia, millet and sorghum. Honeycrisp or Granny Smith apples are good for this, but you can use any baking apple you enjoy eating.

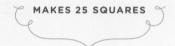

MAKES 25 SQUARES

3 cups (750 mL) peeled, chopped fresh apples

½ cup (125 mL) raisins

⅓ cup (75 mL) organic cane sugar

1 ½ Tbsp (22 mL) cornstarch

½ tsp (2 mL) cinnamon

¼ tsp (1 mL) salt

pinch nutmeg

1 Tbsp (15 mL) ground chia seeds

¼ cup (60 mL) boiling water

¾ cup (175 mL) oat flour

¾ cup (175 mL) sorghum flour

½ cup (125 mL) millet flour

½ cup (125 mL) tapioca starch

2 ¼ cups (550 mL) large-flake, old-fashioned oats

½ cup (125 mL) lightly packed brown sugar

1 cup (250 mL) unsalted butter, melted

1 Tbsp (15 mL) liquid honey

Lightly spray or grease a 9-inch (2.5 L) square baking pan. Line the bottom with parchment paper. Preheat the oven to 350°F (180°C).

Place the apples, raisins, cane sugar, cornstarch, cinnamon, salt and nutmeg in a large saucepan with 1 cup (250 mL) of water and bring to a boil. Turn down to a simmer and cook for 3 to 5 minutes, until the mixture begins to thicken. Remove from the heat and set aside to cool completely in the saucepan.

Combine the chia with the boiling water in a small bowl. Gently stir with a fork to ensure the ground seeds are evenly distributed. Set aside to thicken for about 10 minutes.

Whisk together the oat, sorghum and millet flours, tapioca starch, oats and brown sugar with a pinch of salt. Add the chia mixture, melted butter and honey and mix everything together. Divide this mixture into two portions. Press one half firmly into the prepared pan to make a base. Spread the apple-raisin mixture evenly overtop. Add the remaining oat mixture on top, pressing down lightly with your hands.

Bake for 25 minutes. Remove from the oven and allow to cool completely in the pan. Chill for at least 2 hours, cut into 25 squares and serve.

PER SERVING: Energy 180 calories; Protein 3 g; Carbohydrates 24 g; Dietary Fiber 2 g; Fat 8 g; Sugar 9 g; Cholesterol 20 mg; Sodium 30 mg

STORAGE

Refrigerator: airtight container, 10 days

Hawaiian Oat Squares

A no-bake square made with oats (or any other flakes), virgin coconut oil and dried fruit! Customize this with any other fruit or nuts you like. This recipe uses a coconut oil and butter combination rather than all coconut oil for the best flavor. This is a great pocket snack!

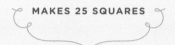

MAKES 25 SQUARES

Lightly grease or spray with cooking oil an 8-inch (2 L) square baking pan. Line the bottom and sides with one piece of parchment, big enough so that it can fold over itself to completely cover the top of the pan.

Place the coconut oil, butter, honey and brown sugar in a medium saucepan. Bring to a boil and boil for 1 minute. Remove from the heat and stir in the vanilla. Set aside to cool.

Mix together the oats (or other flakes), pineapple, papaya, coconut and chia in a large bowl.

Pour the syrup mixture over the oat flake mixture. Stir until everything is combined and the mixture is evenly moistened. Press the mixture firmly and evenly into the pan, folding in the side pieces of parchment to cover the mixture and keep your hands clean.

Chill in the pan for 2 hours. Remove from the pan and cut into 25 squares.

Store the squares separated by layers of wax paper or parchment.

PER SERVING: Energy 120 calories; Protein 2 g; Carbohydrates 15 g; Dietary Fiber 2 g; Fat 6 g; Sugar 7 g; Cholesterol 5 mg; Sodium 0 mg

¼ cup (60 mL) virgin coconut oil

¼ cup (60 mL) unsalted butter

¼ cup (60 mL) liquid honey or pure maple syrup

¼ cup (60 mL) lightly packed brown sugar

2 tsp (10 mL) pure vanilla extract

3 cups (750 mL) quick oats (or chopped old-fashioned oats, millet, quinoa or buckwheat flakes)

⅓ cup (75 mL) chopped dried pineapple

⅓ cup (75 mL) chopped dried papaya

⅓ cup (75 mL) unsweetened medium-shredded coconut

1 Tbsp (15 mL) chia seeds

STORAGE

Refrigerator: airtight container, 10 days

White Chocolate, Orange and Nut Butter Quinoa Squares

This simple no-bake square made with quinoa puffs has the fresh flavor of oranges and the sweetness of white chocolate and maple syrup.

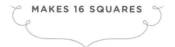

MAKES 16 SQUARES

1 Tbsp (15 mL) ground chia seeds

¼ cup (60 mL) fresh orange juice

1 tsp (5 mL) orange zest

1 cup (250 mL) unsalted smooth peanut or almond butter

½ cup (125 mL) pure maple syrup

¼ cup (60 mL) virgin coconut oil

1 cup (250 mL) white chocolate chips

3 cups (750 mL) quinoa puffs

1 cup (250 mL) unsweetened shredded coconut

¾ cup (175 mL) dried sweetened cranberries or chopped dried cherries

½ cup (125 mL) chopped almonds

Lightly spray or grease an 8-inch (2 L) square pan. Line the bottom and sides with one piece of parchment, big enough so that it can fold over itself to completely cover the top of the pan.

Combine the chia, orange juice and zest in a small bowl. Gently stir with a fork to ensure the ground seeds are evenly distributed. Set aside to thicken, at least 10 minutes.

In a large saucepan over medium-low heat, combine the peanut butter, maple syrup and coconut oil. Stir until smooth and well combined.

Mix in the chocolate chips, stirring until melted. Remove from the heat and add the chia mixture. Stir the puffs, coconut, cranberries and almonds into the chocolate mixture until evenly combined. Press the mixture firmly and evenly into the pan, folding in the side pieces of parchment to cover the mixture and keep your hands clean.

Cool for at least 1 hour in the refrigerator then cut into squares and enjoy.

PER SERVING: Energy 190 calories; Protein 4 g; Carbohydrates 18 g; Dietary Fiber 2 g; Fat 13 g; Sugar 11 g; Cholesterol 0 mg; Sodium 10 mg

BAKING TIP
Try using millet or buckwheat puffs instead of quinoa puffs, or try a combination of puffs.

STORAGE
Refrigerator: airtight container, 1 week

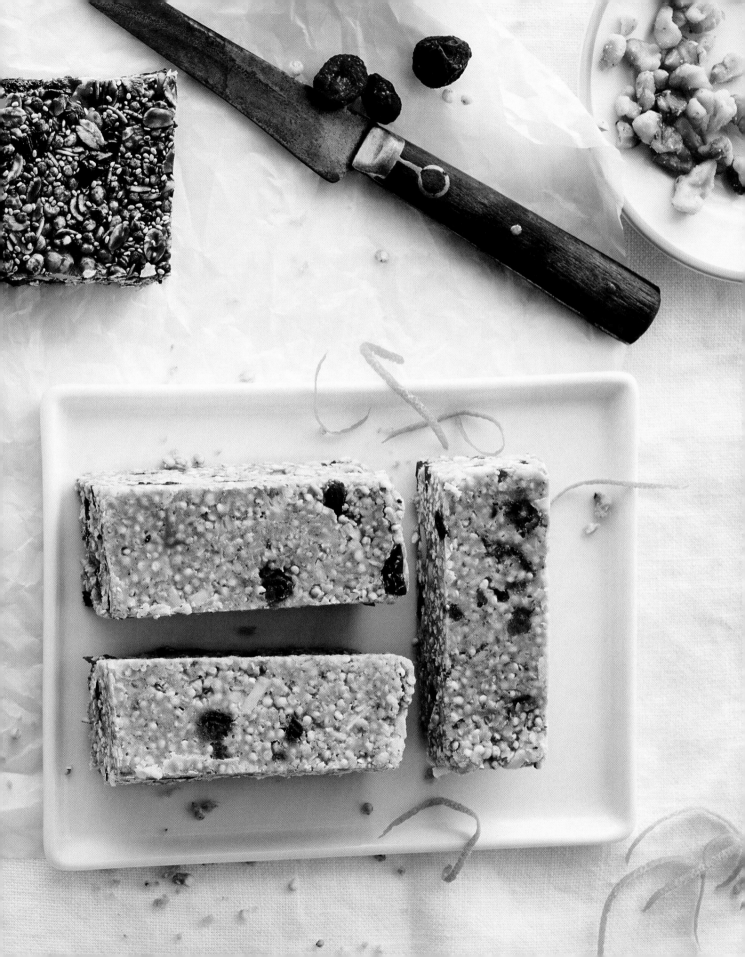

Chocolate Fruit and Nut Chia Squares

These no-bake squares are thick and chewy. Loaded with the fruit and nut flavors of coconut, hazelnuts and raisins, they also have the goodness of quinoa, oats and chia. This is a great portable snack for taking on a hike, keeping in the car, taking along to your workout or giving to the kids after school.

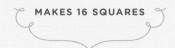

MAKES 16 SQUARES

1 Tbsp (15 mL) ground chia seeds

¼ cup (60 mL) boiling water or hot coffee

1 cup (250 mL) large-flake, old-fashioned oats

1 cup (250 mL) quinoa flakes (or millet or buckwheat flakes)

1 cup (250 mL) unsweetened shredded coconut

¾ cup (175 mL) chopped hazelnuts

1 cup (250 mL) almond butter (crunchy or smooth)

½ cup (125 mL) pure maple syrup

¼ cup (60 mL) virgin coconut oil

1 cup (250 mL) semisweet chocolate chips

1 tsp (5 mL) pure vanilla extract

⅓ cup (75 mL) seedless raisins

Line a rimmed baking sheet with parchment paper. Lightly spray or grease an 8-inch (2 L) square pan. Line the bottom and sides with one piece of parchment, big enough so that it can fold over itself to completely cover the top of the pan. Preheat the oven to 350°F (180°C).

Combine the chia with the boiling water or coffee in a small bowl. Gently stir with a fork to ensure the ground seeds are evenly distributed. Set aside to thicken, at least 10 minutes.

Evenly spread the oats, flakes, coconut and hazelnuts on the prepared rimmed baking sheet. Toast in the oven for 5 to 6 minutes, mixing it at intervals, until most of the mixture is toasted and fragrant. Set aside to cool briefly on the baking pan.

In a large saucepan over medium-low heat, combine the almond butter, maple syrup and coconut oil. Stir until smooth and well combined. (If the mixture is slightly lumpy, blend it with an electric mixer or immersion blender to smooth it out.) Add the chocolate chips and stir until melted. Remove from the heat and add the vanilla and the chia mixture. Stir the oats, flakes, coconut, hazelnuts and raisins into the chocolate mixture until evenly combined. Press the mixture firmly and evenly into the pan, folding in the side pieces of parchment to cover the mixture and keep your hands clean.

Cool for 1 hour in the refrigerator. Remove from the pan and cut into 16 squares.

PER SERVING: Energy 210 calories; Protein 4 g; Carbohydrates 19 g; Dietary Fiber 3 g; Fat 13 g; Sugar 9 g; Cholesterol 0 mg; Sodium 45 mg

BAKING TIP
For an even stronger mocha flavor, add an additional 1 Tbsp (15 mL) of instant coffee to the hot chia mixture (even if you're using coffee instead of water).

STORAGE
Room Temperature: airtight container, 10 days

Chocolate, Walnut and Prune Millet Quinoa Squares

A chewy chocolate fruit and nut bar that may remind you of a certain popular candy bar — but this one tastes better, and it's a healthier option, too.

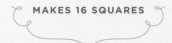

MAKES 16 SQUARES

Line a rimmed baking sheet with parchment paper. Lightly grease or spray with cooking oil an 8-inch (2 L) square cake pan. Line the bottom and sides with one piece of parchment, big enough so that it can fold over itself to completely cover the top of the pan. Preheat the oven to 350°F (180°C).

Evenly spread the oats, walnuts and chia seeds on the baking sheet. Place in the oven to toast for 5 to 6 minutes, until fragrant. Remove from the oven and set aside to cool briefly in the pan.

In a large bowl, mix together the quinoa puffs, millet puffs and prunes. Add the toasted oats, walnuts and chia seeds. Stir and set aside.

In a medium saucepan, stir the sugar and cocoa with the honey, maple syrup, butter and salt. Bring to a boil and then turn down the heat to a simmer. Cook until the butter is melted and the sugar is dissolved completely, 3 to 4 minutes. Remove from the heat, then stir in the vanilla and cinnamon.

Pour the syrup mixture over the puff mixture. Stir until blended and the mixture is evenly moistened. Press the mixture firmly and evenly into the pan, folding in the side pieces of parchment to cover the mixture and keep your hands clean.

Chill in the pan for 2 hours. Remove from the pan using the parchment paper and cut into squares. Best served cold.

Store the squares separated by layers of wax paper or parchment.

PER SERVING: Energy 180 calories; Protein 3 g; Carbohydrates 23 g; Dietary Fiber 3 g; Fat 9 g; Sugar 12 g; Cholesterol 10 mg; Sodium 40 mg

1 cup (250 mL) old-fashioned rolled oats

1 cup (250 mL) chopped walnuts

1/3 cup (75 mL) chia seeds

1 cup (250 mL) quinoa puffs

1 cup (250 mL) millet puffs

3/4 cup (175 mL) chopped, pitted dried prunes

1/2 cup (125 mL) lightly packed brown sugar

1/4 cup (60 mL) unsweetened cocoa powder

1/4 cup (60 mL) liquid honey

1/4 cup (60 mL) pure maple syrup

1/4 cup (60 mL) unsalted butter

1/4 tsp (1 mL) salt

1 tsp (5 mL) pure vanilla extract

1/2 tsp (2 mL) cinnamon

STORAGE

Refrigerator: airtight container, 10 days

BAKING TIP

· Try using buckwheat or amaranth puffs instead of quinoa or millet puffs, or try a combination of puffs.

· Maximize your antioxidants by avoiding Dutch process cocoa and using regular unsweetened cocoa powder.

Cranberry Lemon Millet Quinoa Squares

This tasty no-bake bar is loaded with lemon flavor and is delightfully chewy. Using both quinoa and millet puffs gives it additional texture — but if you just have one or the other, use 2 cups (500 mL) of either one.

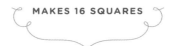

MAKES 16 SQUARES

1 cup (250 mL) old-fashioned rolled oats

½ cup (125 mL) chopped almonds

⅓ cup (75 mL) chia seeds

1 cup (250 mL) millet puffs

1 cup (250 mL) quinoa puffs

½ cup (125 mL) dried sweetened cranberries (chopped if they are larger sized)

½ cup (125 mL) lightly packed brown sugar

¼ cup (60 mL) liquid honey

¼ cup (60 mL) pure maple syrup

¼ cup (60 mL) unsalted butter

¼ tsp (1 mL) salt

2 tsp (10 mL) fresh lemon juice

2 tsp (10 mL) lemon zest

Line a rimmed baking sheet with parchment paper. Lightly grease or spray with cooking oil an 8-inch (2 L) square cake pan. Line the bottom and sides with one piece of parchment, big enough so that it can fold over itself to completely cover the top of the pan. Preheat the oven to 350°F (180°C).

Evenly spread the oats, almonds and chia seeds on the rimmed baking sheet. Place in the oven to toast for 5 to 6 minutes, until fragrant. Remove from the oven and set aside to cool briefly on the baking tray.

In a large bowl, mix together the millet and quinoa puffs and dried cranberries. Add the toasted almonds, oats and chia seeds. Stir and set aside.

In a medium saucepan, stir the sugar with the honey, maple syrup, butter and salt. Bring to a boil and turn down the heat to a simmer. Cook, stirring frequently, until the butter is melted and the sugar is dissolved completely, 3 to 4 minutes. Remove from the heat and stir in the lemon juice and zest.

Pour the syrup mixture over the puff mixture. Stir until all the ingredients are fully blended and the mixture is evenly moistened. Press the mixture firmly and evenly into the pan, folding in the side pieces of parchment to cover the mixture and keep your hands clean.

Chill in the pan for 2 hours. Remove from the pan and cut into squares. Best served cold.

Store the squares separated by layers of wax paper or parchment.

PER SERVING: Energy 150 calories; Protein 3 g; Carbohydrates 23 g; Dietary Fiber 2 g; Fat 6 g; Sugar 10 g; Cholesterol 10 mg; Sodium 40 mg

BAKING TIP
Try using buckwheat puffs instead of quinoa puffs, or use a combination of puffs.

STORAGE
Room Temperature: **airtight container, 10 days**

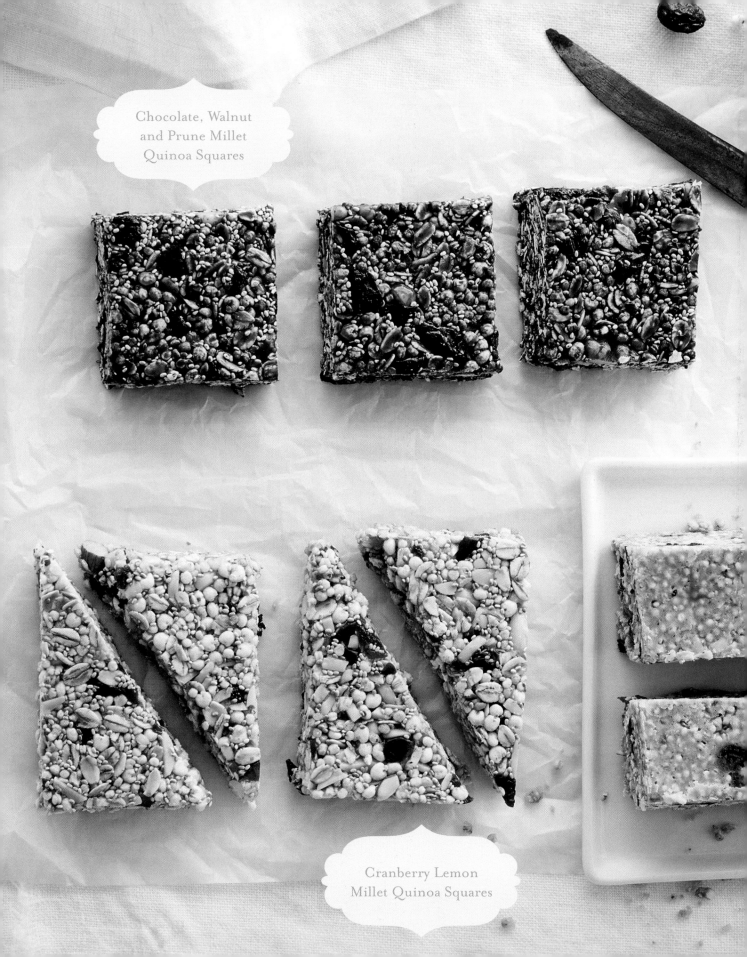

Chocolate, Walnut
and Prune Millet
Quinoa Squares

Cranberry Lemon
Millet Quinoa Squares

Espresso Cookie Bars with Honey Marshmallow Meringue

*This cookie bar made with sorghum and teff flour has chocolate and marshmallow
as treat ingredients with the added luxurious flavor of coffee.*

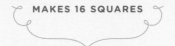

MAKES 16 SQUARES

⅓ cup (75 mL) sorghum flour

⅓ cup (75 mL) teff flour

⅓ cup (75 mL) tapioca starch

2 Tbsp (30 mL) instant espresso
coffee powder

⅓ cup (75 mL) unsalted butter,
softened

½ cup (125 mL) organic
cane sugar

1 large egg

⅔ cup (150 mL) semisweet
chocolate chips

3 large egg whites, at room
temperature

¼ tsp (1 mL) cream of tartar

pinch salt

1 Tbsp (15 mL) liquid honey

½ tsp (2 mL) pure vanilla extract

Lightly spray or grease an 8-inch (2 L) square pan. Line the pan
with parchment paper. Preheat the oven to 350°F (180°C).

Whisk together the sorghum and teff flours, tapioca starch and
espresso powder. Set aside. Cream the butter with the sugar
and egg in a medium bowl. Add the butter mixture to the flour
mixture, stirring until well combined. Pour the mixture into
the prepared pan. Evenly scatter the chocolate chips on top of the
batter. Set aside.

In a separate medium bowl, beat the egg whites, cream of tartar
and salt with the honey and vanilla until very stiff peaks form.
Evenly spread this marshmallow mixture over the chocolate chips
in the pan.

Bake for 20 to 25 minutes, until the top of the marshmallow
meringue is an even golden color. Cool in the pan and cut
into squares.

PER SERVING: Energy 130 calories; Protein 2 g; Carbohydrates 18 g;
Dietary Fiber 1 g; Fat 6 g; Sugar 11 g; Cholesterol 20 mg; Sodium 35 mg

STORAGE

Refrigerator: **airtight container, 1 week**

Milk Chocolate and Orange Blondies

These chewy milk chocolate—topped blondies have a complementary hint of orange. Almond butter gives them added nutty flavor.

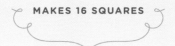

MAKES 16 SQUARES

Lightly grease an 8-inch (2 L) square cake pan. Line the pan with parchment paper. Preheat the oven to 350°F (180°C).

Cream the almond butter and unsalted butter in a medium bowl. Beat in the brown sugar, eggs, vanilla and orange zest until smooth. Set aside.

In a separate small bowl, whisk together the flour, baking powder and salt. Add the flour mixture to the almond butter mixture. Spread the batter evenly in the prepared pan.

Bake for 18 to 20 minutes, or until a toothpick inserted in the center comes out with just a few crumbs. Do not overbake.

Melt the chocolate chips (in a microwave oven or double boiler) and spoon into a small resealable plastic bag. Cut ¼ inch (0.5 cm) from one corner and pipe the chocolate onto the blondies. Let cool in the pan for 15 minutes before cutting into 16 squares.

PER SERVING: Energy 180 calories; Protein 4 g; Carbohydrates 15 g; Dietary Fiber 2 g; Fat 12 g; Sugar 9 g; Cholesterol 30 mg; Sodium 55 mg

¾ cup (175 mL) almond or hazelnut butter (smooth or crunchy)

¼ cup (60 mL) unsalted butter, softened

¾ cup (175 mL) lightly packed brown sugar

2 large eggs

1 ½ tsp (7 mL) pure vanilla extract

½ tsp (2 mL) orange zest

¾ cup (175 mL) millet flour

1 tsp (5 mL) baking powder

¼ tsp (1 mL) salt

⅓ cup (75 mL) milk chocolate chips

STORAGE
Refrigerator: **airtight container, 10 days**

Praline Cheesecake Blondies

Delicious, sweet and creamy, these praline squares are made with sorghum and millet. They are perfect when you want a decadent treat, combining caramel, the toasty flavor of almond butter and delectable cream cheese.

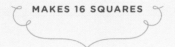

MAKES 16 SQUARES

BASE

¼ cup (60 mL) unsalted butter

¾ cup (175 mL) almond butter (smooth or crunchy)

2 large eggs

¾ cup (175 mL) lightly packed brown sugar

2 tsp (10 mL) pure vanilla extract

½ cup (125 mL) sorghum flour

¼ cup (60 mL) millet flour

1 tsp (5 mL) baking powder

¼ tsp (1 mL) salt

¾ cup (175 mL) chopped pecans

CHEESECAKE

8 oz (225 g) package cream cheese, softened

¼ cup (60 mL) organic cane sugar

1 large egg

1 tsp (5 mL) pure vanilla extract

2 tsp (10 mL) sorghum flour

CARAMEL

2 Tbsp (30 mL) unsalted butter

½ cup (125 mL) lightly packed brown sugar

¼ cup (60 mL) 5% cream

1 tsp (5 mL) pure vanilla extract

Lightly grease an 8-inch (2 L) square baking pan. Line the bottom with parchment paper. Preheat the oven to 350°F (180°C).

For the base, cream both butters together in a medium bowl. Beat in the eggs, sugar and vanilla. Set aside. In a separate medium bowl, whisk together the sorghum and millet flours, baking powder and salt. Add the butter mixture to the flour mixture. Mix well then add the pecans. Spread evenly into the prepared pan. Set aside.

For the cheesecake, in a medium bowl, beat the cream cheese, sugar, egg and vanilla. Mix in the flour. Spread this mixture over the almond base in the pan. Set aside.

For the caramel, in a medium saucepan over medium heat, whisk the butter with the brown sugar and cream. Bring to a boil and then turn down the heat to a simmer. Simmer for 7 minutes, whisking constantly. Remove from the heat and stir in the vanilla. Let cool slightly. Pour this caramel over the cheesecake filling and swirl the surface of the cheesecake with a knife until the desired pattern is achieved.

Bake for 30 to 35 minutes, until a toothpick comes out with just a few crumbs. Allow to cool completely in the pan then refrigerate for at least 2 hours or overnight. Cut into squares. Serve cold.

PER SERVING: Energy 300 calories; Protein 6 g; Carbohydrates 23 g; Dietary Fiber 2 g; Fat 21 g; Sugar 16 g; Cholesterol 65 mg; Sodium 100 mg

STORAGE

Refrigerator: airtight container, 1 week

Chocolate Hazelnut Brownies

Made with teff and hazelnut butter, these brownies are moist and full
of luxurious chocolate hazelnut flavor — and guaranteed to impress.

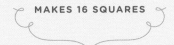

MAKES 16 SQUARES

Lightly spray with cooking oil or grease an 8-inch (2 L) square cake pan. Line the pan with parchment paper. Preheat the oven to 350°F (180°C).

In a medium bowl, cream the hazelnut and unsalted butter. Beat in the brown sugar, eggs and vanilla until smooth.

In a separate small bowl, whisk together the flour, cocoa, baking powder and salt. Mix this into the hazelnut butter mixture. Spread the batter evenly into the prepared pan.

Spoon the chocolate hazelnut spread into a small resealable plastic bag. Cut ¼ inch (1 cm) off one corner. Pipe five horizontal lines equal distances apart. Take a toothpick and make 8 to 10 perpendicular lines running back and forth to create arrow designs on the top of the batter.

Bake for 18 to 20 minutes, or until a toothpick inserted in the center comes out with just a few crumbs. Do not overbake. Let cool in the pan for 15 minutes before cutting into 16 squares.

PER SERVING: Energy 170 calories; Protein 3 g; Carbohydrates 16 g; Dietary Fiber 2 g; Fat 11 g; Sugar 10 g; Cholesterol 30 mg; Sodium 50 mg

¾ cup (175 mL) hazelnut or almond butter (smooth or crunchy)

¼ cup (60 mL) unsalted butter, softened

¾ cup (175 mL) lightly packed brown sugar

2 large eggs

1 ½ tsp (7 mL) pure vanilla extract

½ cup (125 mL) teff flour

⅓ cup (75 mL) unsweetened cocoa powder

1 tsp (5 mL) baking powder

¼ tsp (1 mL) salt

⅓ cup (75 mL) chocolate hazelnut spread

STORAGE
Room Temperature: airtight container, 1 week
Refrigerator: airtight container, 1 week

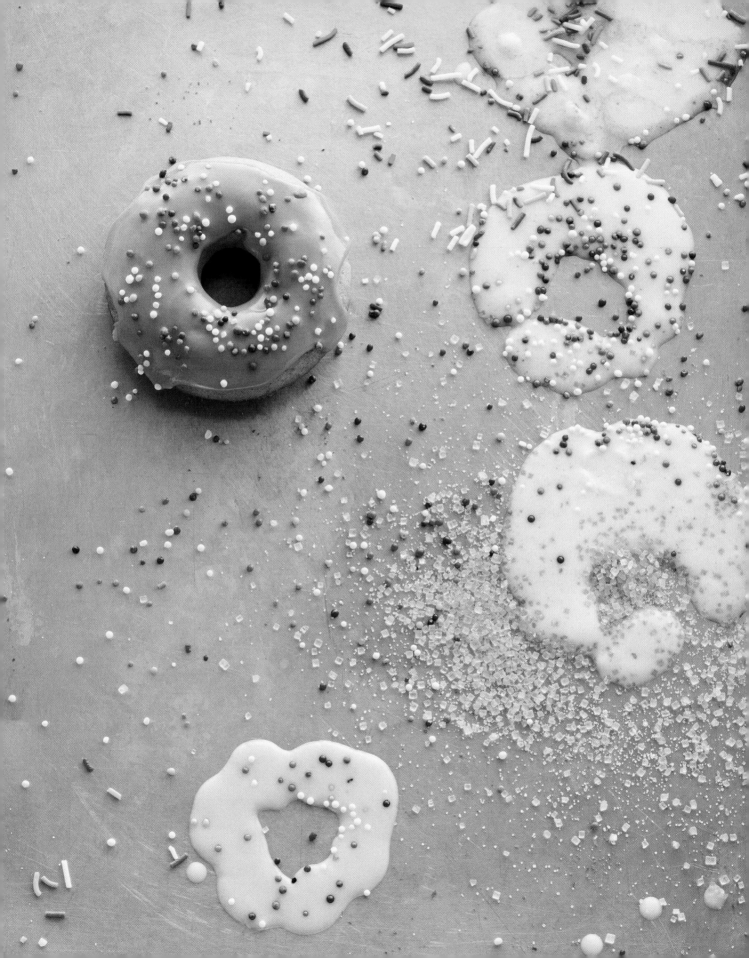

Cakes, Loaves, Muffins and More

Graham-Style Wafers   46

Thyme, Rosemary
and Parmesan Oatcakes   49

Cranberry Lemon Oatcakes   50

Mint Cherry Country Baked Biscuits   51

Light and Fluffy Cream Puffs   52

Golden Buttermilk Biscuits   54

Parmesan Salt and Pepper Biscuits   55

Toffee Maple Bacon Scones   56

Cranberry, Walnut and
Rosemary Muffins   58

Strawberry Jam Oat Muffins   59

Sweet Potato Muffins   60

Wild Blueberry Buttermilk
Bran Muffins   61

Nut and Chocolate Muffins   62

Almond Ancient Grain Cupcakes   63

Honey Ginger Carrot Cakes with
Lime Cream Cheese Frosting   64

Old-Fashioned Cake Doughnuts   67

Double Chocolate Cake Doughnuts   68

Banana Breakfast Bread   70

Breakfast Popover Loaf   71

Prune Spice Loaf   72

Chocolate Swirl Banana Loaf   73

Maple Raisin Cinnamon Buns   74

Raspberry Lemon Quinoa
and Oat Loaves   76

Mint Chocolate–Dipped
Cake Bites   77

Mini Maple Cherry Cheesecakes   79

Ancient Grain Pound Cake   80

Ancient Grain Angel Food Cake   81

Fluffy White Quinoa Cake   82

Cinnamon Apple Coffee Cake   83

Coconut Cake with
Whipped Yogurt Frosting   84

Lemon Crêpe Cake   86

Chocolate Cream Cheese
Coconut Cake   88

Devil's Food Cake   90

Outrageous Quinoa
Chocolate Cake   91

Blackberry Honey Clafoutis   94

Raisin Farmhouse Pudding   95

Pineapple Citrus Berry Crisp   96

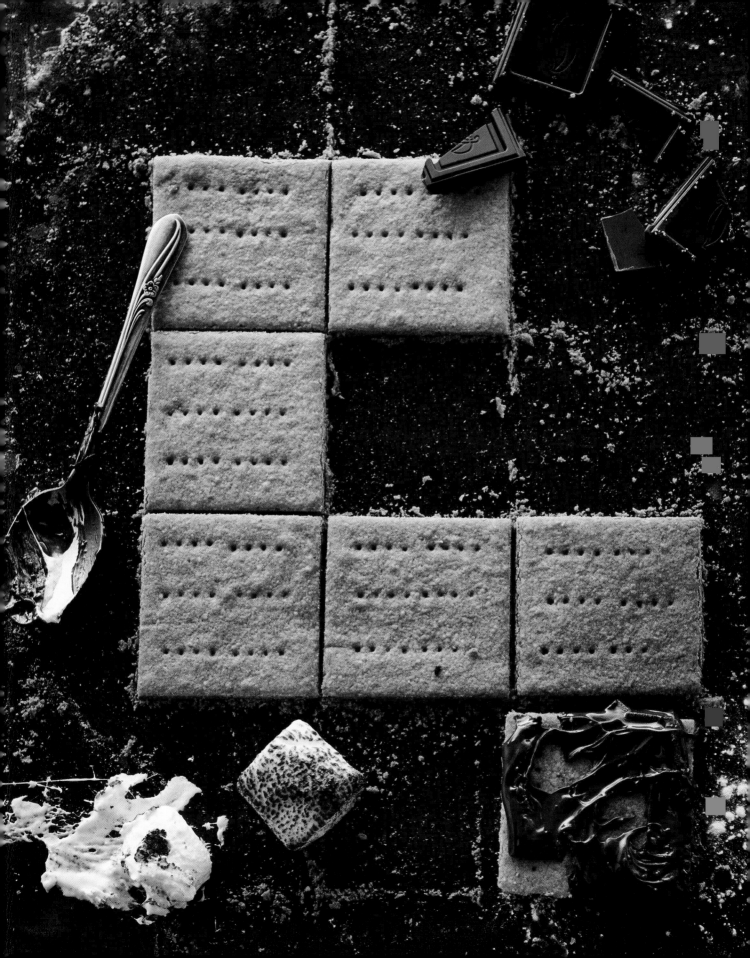

Sometimes it's the little things that make a person's day. Many beloved family recipes are simple baked goods. Sweet and warm muffins, cakes, loaves and biscuits have long been staples in North America and Europe and in many a kitchen across the globe. Despite many simple baked goods being originally based on traditional flours containing gluten, it is not impossible to make countless classics gluten-free, including campfire s'mores, healthy muffins or fluffy scones for breakfast or tea. The evolution of these great favorites continues as we modify them to meet dietary requirements, use new ingredients and basically answer the call of our creative cooking minds.

Haven't had graham wafers in years? Try our gluten-free Graham-Style Wafers (page 46); they won't disappoint you! Need savory options? Try Parmesan Salt and Pepper Biscuits (page 55), or add your favorite fixings to the Golden Buttermilk Biscuits (page 54). Try angel food cake reinvented in our Ancient Grain Angel Food Cake (page 81), or for a uniquely impressive treat, try Toffee Maple Bacon Scones (page 56). Old-Fashioned Cake Doughnuts (page 67) and Double Chocolate Cake Doughnuts (page 68) make great weekday snacks, and teatime and takeaway treats. For heartier bits you can serve to guests or offer for dessert, try the Lemon Crêpe Cake (page 86), Coconut Cake with Whipped Yogurt Frosting (page 84) or the guaranteed-to-please Outrageous Quinoa Chocolate Cake (page 91).

Graham-Style Wafers

This is the real graham wafer! If you've been living without graham wafers because of gluten, then you're in for a treat! This makes a delicious graham crust option for both pies and squares, and even for those popular fireside s'mores! Use as a tasty gluten-free replacement wherever graham wafers are normally used.

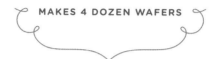

MAKES 4 DOZEN WAFERS

1 ½ cups (375 mL) potato starch, plus additional for rolling

1 cup (250 mL) oat flour

⅓ cup (75 mL) oat bran

1 Tbsp (15 mL) psyllium husks

1 ½ tsp (7 mL) baking powder

½ tsp (2 mL) baking soda

½ tsp (2 mL) salt

⅔ cup (150 mL) unsalted butter, softened

½ cup (125 mL) lightly packed brown sugar

¼ cup (60 mL) liquid honey

2 tsp (10 mL) pure vanilla extract

Combine the potato starch, oat flour, oat bran, psyllium, baking powder, baking soda and salt in a medium bowl. Whisk together until evenly combined, then set aside.

In a separate large bowl, beat the butter and brown sugar together until smooth. Add the honey and vanilla and mix well. Add the dry ingredients in four additions, mixing until fully combined. Divide the dough into two balls, flatten them into disks, wrap in plastic wrap and chill in the refrigerator for 1 hour (or more). When the dough is removed from the refrigerator, manipulate it with your hands to soften it slightly if it's too hard to roll.

Cut a piece of parchment paper to fit the size of one large or two small baking sheets, then remove the parchment from the baking sheet and dust it with flour. Preheat the oven to 350°F (180°C).

Place the dough on the parchment paper, dust it slightly with flour and use a rolling pin to roll it to ¼ inch (0.5 cm) thick, turning and dusting occasionally. Use a pizza cutter to cut wafers 2 ½ inches (6 cm) square. Leave the cut dough intact (do not separate the cut squares) on the parchment and place it on the baking sheet. Prick each square of dough with a fork two or three times in its center. Bake for 15 minutes, or until the edge of the dough is slightly golden. Remove from the oven and re-cut the squares with the pizza cutter while still warm. Allow to cool completely on the baking sheet.

PER SERVING: Energy 70 calories; Protein 0 g; Carbohydrates 10 g; Dietary Fiber 1 g; Fat 3 g; Sugar 3 g; Cholesterol 5 mg; Sodium 40 mg

BAKING TIP
Use cookie cutters to make wafers in a variety of fun shapes.

STORAGE
Room Temperature: airtight container, 1 week

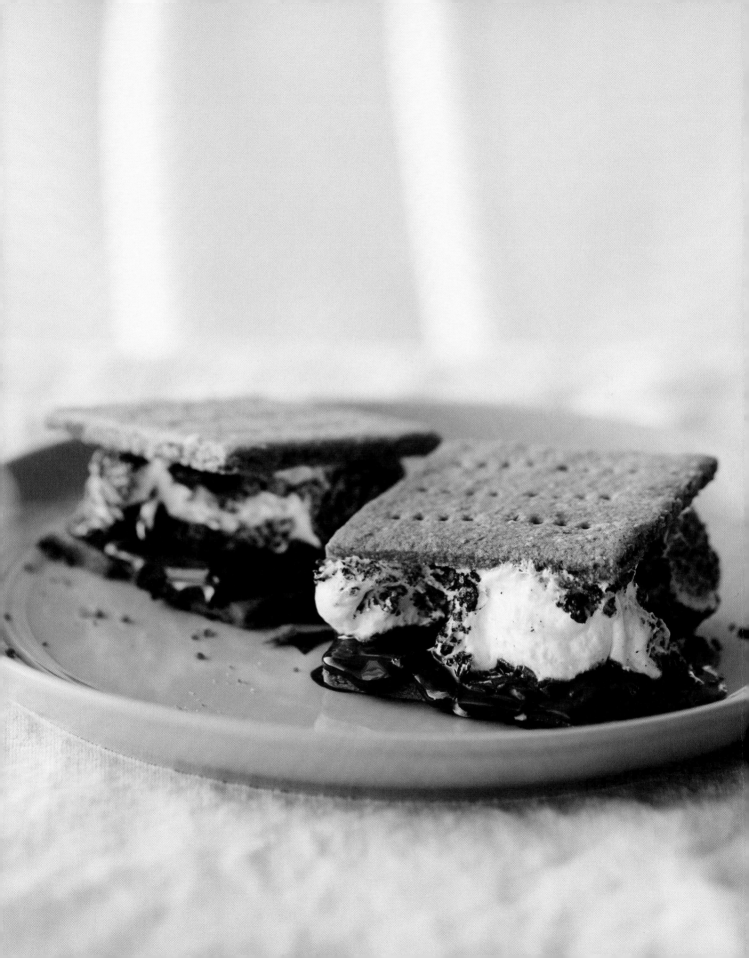

Switch up the flavor with other herb combinations
such as Parmesan cheese with oregano, chives or parsley.

Room Temperature: airtight container or bag, 1 week
Freezer: airtight freezer bag or container, 1 month

Thyme, Rosemary and Parmesan Oatcakes

An oatcake is a dense flatbread biscuit, like a softer cracker. Although traditionally cooked on a griddle, this version is baked (like the Cranberry Lemon Oatcakes on page 50). The oatcakes are great served alongside a light lunch, soups and stews or even just a selection of fruit and cheese.

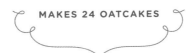

MAKES 24 OATCAKES

Lightly spray with cooking oil or grease a large baking sheet. Line the baking sheet with parchment paper. Preheat the oven to 350°F (180°C).

Add the chia to ¼ cup (60 mL) of the boiling water in a small bowl. Gently stir it with a fork to ensure the ground seeds are evenly distributed. Set aside to thicken, about 10 minutes.

Whisk together the oat flour, salt and baking soda in a medium bowl. Add the thyme, rosemary and Parmesan. Mix in the remaining ½ cup (125 mL) of boiling water, the chia mixture and melted butter. Use your hands to roll this mixture into a dough. Shape the dough into 1 ½- to 2-inch (4–5 cm) balls and place them on the prepared baking sheet ¼ inch (0.5 cm) apart. Flatten each one with the palm of your hand.

Bake for 20 to 22 minutes, until the edges are golden. Remove the oatcakes from the sheet to cool completely on a rack.

PER SERVING: Energy 35 calories; Protein 1 g; Carbohydrates 4 g; Dietary Fiber 1 g; Fat 1 g; Sugar 0 g; Cholesterol 0 mg; Sodium 40 mg

1 Tbsp (15 mL) ground chia seeds

¾ cup (185 mL) boiling water

2 cups (500 mL) oat flour

¼ tsp (1 mL) salt

¼ tsp (1 mL) baking soda

1 Tbsp (15 mL) chopped fresh thyme leaves

1 Tbsp (15 mL) chopped fresh rosemary

1 Tbsp (15 mL) grated Parmesan cheese

1 Tbsp (15 mL) melted butter

Cranberry Lemon Oatcakes

An oatcake is a dense flatbread biscuit, like a softer cracker. Although traditionally cooked on a griddle, this version is baked (like the Thyme, Rosemary and Parmesan Oatcakes on page 49), and is sweetened with honey and fresh lemon zest. These are great served alongside a light lunch, fruit and cheese or tea.

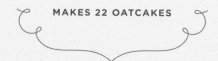

MAKES 22 OATCAKES

1 Tbsp (15 mL) ground chia seeds

¾ cup (185 mL) boiling water

2 cups (500 mL) oat flour

¼ tsp (1 mL) salt

¼ tsp (1 mL) baking soda

½ cup (125 mL) chopped, dried sweetened cranberries

2 tsp (10 mL) lemon zest

1 Tbsp (15 mL) melted unsalted butter

1 Tbsp (15 mL) liquid honey

Lightly spray with cooking oil or grease a large baking sheet. Line the baking sheet with parchment paper. Preheat the oven to 350°F (180°C).

Place the chia in ¼ cup (60 mL) of the boiling water in a small bowl. Gently stir with a fork to ensure the ground seeds are evenly distributed. Set aside to thicken, about 10 minutes.

Whisk together the oat flour, salt and baking soda in a medium bowl. Add the cranberries and lemon zest. Mix in the remaining ½ cup (125 mL) boiling water, the chia mixture, melted butter and honey. Use your hands to roll the mixture into a dough. Shape the dough into 1 ½- to 2-inch (4–5 cm) balls and place them on the prepared baking sheet ¼ inch (1 cm) apart. Flatten each one with the palm of your hand.

Bake for 20 to 22 minutes, until the edges are golden. Remove the oatcakes from the sheet to cool completely on a rack.

PER SERVING: Energy 45 calories; Protein 1 g; Carbohydrates 8 g; Dietary Fiber 1 g; Fat 1 g; Sugar 3 g; Cholesterol 0 mg; Sodium 40 mg

STORAGE

Room Temperature: airtight container or bag, 1 week

Freezer: airtight freezer bag or container, 1 month

Mint Cherry Country Baked Biscuits

Tender, flaky sorghum, oat and coconut flour biscuits are baked on top of sweet summer cherries and fresh mint in this recipe. A terrific brunch dish that begs to be eaten alfresco!

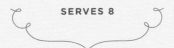

SERVES 8

Lightly spray with cooking oil or grease a 9- × 13-inch (3.5 L) casserole dish. Preheat the oven to 425°F (220°C).

Add the chia to the boiling water in a small bowl. Gently stir with a fork to ensure the ground seeds are evenly distributed. Set aside to thicken, about 10 minutes.

Place the cherries and ⅓ cup (75 mL) sugar in a medium sauce-pan with ¾ cup (175 mL) of water and bring to a boil over high heat. Turn down the heat to medium-low and simmer, uncovered, for 5 to 6 minutes, until the sugar is completely dissolved and the cherries have softened. Remove from the heat and stir in the vanilla and 1 Tbsp (15 mL) of the mint. Pour this mixture into the prepared baking dish and set aside.

Place the sorghum, oat and coconut flours, potato starch, arrowroot starch, xanthan gum, baking powder, baking soda, 2 Tbsp (30 mL) sugar and salt in a large bowl. Whisk until evenly mixed. Using a pastry cutter, cut in the butter until the mixture resembles pea-sized crumbles. Stir in the remainder of the mint. Add the chia mixture and pour in the buttermilk. Using a large spoon, fold the mixture until just combined. Spoon the biscuit mixture by heaping tablespoons (20 mL) on top of the cherry mixture.

Bake for 10 to 12 minutes, until the tops of the biscuits are golden. Serve warm.

Best eaten the day you make them.

PER SERVING: Energy 270 calories; Protein 4 g; Carbohydrates 45 g; Dietary Fiber 5 g; Fat 8 g; Sugar 19 g; Cholesterol 15 mg; Sodium 190 mg

1 Tbsp (15 mL) ground chia seeds

¼ cup (60 mL) boiling water

3 cups (750 mL) halved fresh cherries

⅓ cup (75 mL) organic cane sugar

1 ½ tsp (7 mL) vanilla bean paste or pure vanilla extract

3 Tbsp (45 mL) finely chopped fresh mint

⅔ cup (150 mL) sorghum flour

⅓ cup (75 mL) oat flour

⅓ cup (75 mL) coconut flour

⅓ cup (75 mL) potato starch

⅓ cup (75 mL) arrowroot starch

½ tsp (2 mL) xanthan gum

1 Tbsp (15 mL) baking powder

1 tsp (5 mL) baking soda

2 Tbsp (30 mL) organic cane sugar

½ tsp (2 mL) salt

¼ cup (60 mL) cold unsalted butter

¾ cup (175 mL) buttermilk

BAKING TIP
Terrific with whipped cream.

Light and Fluffy Cream Puffs

Whether for brunch, tea or a light dessert, cream puffs are a hit. With this version made with sorghum and rice flours, you'll find it difficult to eat just one. For something a little different, top the whipped cream with your favorite fruit compote (blueberry is good). Another fun option is to add a touch of Irish cream liqueur to the whipped cream.

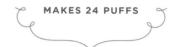

MAKES 24 PUFFS

PUFFS

¼ cup (60 mL) sweet rice flour

3 Tbsp (45 mL) sorghum flour

1 tsp (5 mL) psyllium husks

1 tsp (5 mL) organic cane sugar

pinch salt

¼ cup (60 mL) unsalted butter

2 large eggs, lightly beaten

FILLING

½ cup (125 mL) whipping cream

2 tsp (10 mL) pure maple syrup

½ tsp (2 mL) pure vanilla extract

⅓ cup (75 mL) semisweet
chocolate chips (optional)

powdered (icing) sugar
for dusting (optional,
if not using chocolate)

Line a large baking sheet with parchment paper. Place a medium bowl and a whisk in the refrigerator to chill. Preheat the oven to 400°F (200°C).

For the puffs, whisk together the sweet rice and sorghum flours, psyllium, sugar and salt in a small bowl and set aside. Melt the butter in a medium saucepan with ½ cup (125 mL) of water. Bring to a boil on medium-high heat as the butter melts. Add the flour mixture all at once, stirring vigorously until combined and the dough pulls away from the sides of the saucepan. Cool until the dough is just warm, then use a handheld mixer to beat in the eggs, leaving the dough smooth and thickened. Spoon or pipe the dough in 1-inch (2.5 cm) diameter pieces onto the prepared baking sheet 1 ½ inches (4 cm) apart.

Bake for 15 minutes, until puffed and golden. Remove from the oven and let cool completely on the sheet.

For the filling, take the bowl and whisk from the refrigerator and whip the cream, syrup and vanilla until soft peaks form. Slice each cream puff in half and fill with whipped cream. Melt the chocolate chips in a double boiler or microwave oven (using intervals of 15 seconds until just melted). Let cool slightly, scrape into a resealable plastic bag, snip ⅛ inch (0.3 cm) off one corner and pipe chocolate across the tops of the puffs as desired.

PER SERVING: Energy 50 calories; Protein 1 g; Carbohydrates 3 g; Dietary Fiber 1 g; Fat 4 g; Sugar 1 g; Cholesterol 25 mg; Sodium 20 mg

STORAGE

Room Temperature: **airtight container or bag, 2 days**

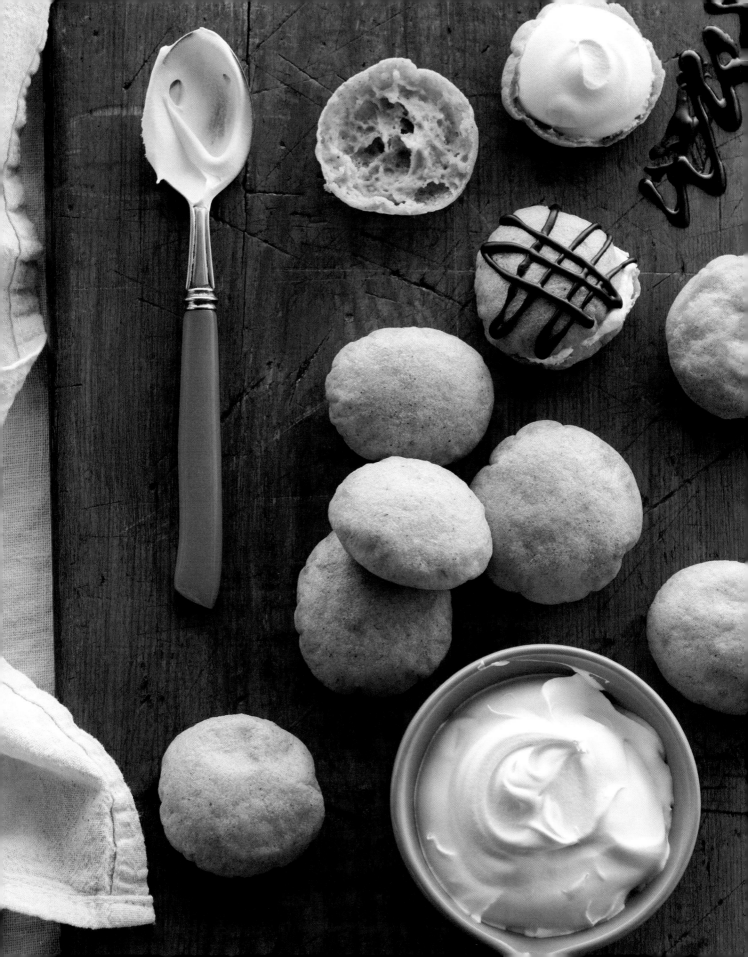

Golden Buttermilk Biscuits

Golden brown on the outside, tender and soft on the inside, these biscuits deliver as good as any conventional biscuits. Make them big enough for breakfast sandwiches, or half the size to serve with breakfast or stew.

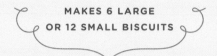

MAKES 6 LARGE OR 12 SMALL BISCUITS

⅔ cup (150 mL) tapioca starch, plus extra for dusting

⅔ cup (150 mL) white rice flour

⅓ cup (75 mL) sorghum flour

1 Tbsp (15 mL) baking powder

1 tsp (5 mL) xanthan gum

½ tsp (2 mL) salt

⅓ cup (75 mL) cold unsalted butter

1 cup (250 mL) buttermilk (or milk-vinegar substitute)

1 ½ tsp (7 mL) unsalted butter, melted

Line a baking sheet with parchment paper.

Whisk together the tapioca starch, rice and sorghum flours, baking powder, xanthan gum and salt in a large bowl. Cut in the cold butter with a pastry cutter or with two knives until the butter is the size of small peas. Pour in the buttermilk and turn the mixture with a spatula until the dough comes together. Turn out onto a floured surface and gently work with your hands until smooth but you can still see pieces of butter. Flour your hands and pat the dough into a square 1 inch (2.5 cm) thick.

Cut the dough into 6 large or 12 small square biscuits. Place the biscuits on the prepared baking sheet at least 1 ½ inches (4 cm) apart. Brush each one with the melted butter and bake for 15 to 17 minutes for the large biscuits and 10 to 12 minutes for the small ones. Remove from the oven and serve warm.

PER SERVING: Energy 220 calories; Protein 3 g; Carbohydrates 26 g; Dietary Fiber 1 g; Fat 11 g; Sugar 3 g; Cholesterol 35 mg; Sodium 210 mg

STORAGE

Room Temperature: airtight container or bag, 3 days

Refrigerator: airtight container or bag, 4 days

Parmesan Salt and Pepper Biscuits

Biscuits hot out of the oven with salty Parmesan and black pepper are perfect to accompany almost any soup, stew or salad. Wrap them in a towel to keep them warm longer.

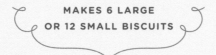

MAKES 6 LARGE OR 12 SMALL BISCUITS

Line a baking sheet with parchment paper.

Whisk together the tapioca starch, rice and sorghum flours, baking powder, xanthan gum, salt and pepper in a large bowl. Stir in ⅓ cup (75 mL) of the Parmesan cheese and the herbs (if using). Cut in the cold butter with a pastry cutter or two knives until the butter is the size of small peas. Pour in the buttermilk and turn the crumbly mixture with a spatula until the dough comes together. Turn out onto a floured surface and gently work with your hands until the dough is smooth but you can still see pieces of butter. Flour your hands and pat the dough into a square 1 inch (2.5 cm) thick.

Cut into 6 large or 12 small square biscuits. Place the biscuits on the prepared baking sheet at least 1 ½ inches (4 cm) apart. Brush each one with the melted butter and sprinkle with the remaining 2 Tbsp (30 mL) of Parmesan. Bake for 15 to 17 minutes for the large biscuits and 10 to 12 minutes for the small biscuits. Remove from the oven and serve warm.

PER SERVING: Energy 290 calories; Protein 6 g; Carbohydrates 35 g; Dietary Fiber 2 g; Fat 14 g; Sugar 2 g; Cholesterol 40 mg; Sodium 210 mg

⅔ cup (150 mL) tapioca starch, plus extra for dusting

⅔ cup (150 mL) white rice flour

⅓ cup (75 mL) sorghum flour

1 Tbsp (15 mL) baking powder

1 tsp (5 mL) xanthan gum

½ tsp (2 mL) salt

¼ tsp (1 mL) freshly ground black pepper

⅓ cup plus 2 Tbsp (75 mL + 30 mL) freshly grated Parmesan cheese

2 Tbsp (30 mL) fresh herbs (chives, dill, parsley) (or 2 tsp/10 mL dried), optional

⅓ cup (75 mL) cold unsalted butter

1 cup (250 mL) cold buttermilk (or cold milk-vinegar substitute)

1 ½ tsp (7 mL) unsalted butter, melted

STORAGE
Room Temperature: airtight container or bag, 3 days
Refrigerator: airtight container or bag, 4 days

Toffee Maple Bacon Scones

Savory meets subtle sweetness in a perfectly fluffy scone with bacon crumbles, toffee bits and a touch of maple. Serve with apple butter.

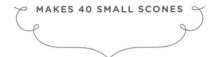

MAKES 40 SMALL SCONES

1 ½ cups (375 mL) tapioca starch

1 ½ cups (375 mL) oat flour

½ cup (125 mL) sorghum flour

5 tsp (25 mL) baking powder

½ tsp (2 mL) salt

¾ cup (175 mL) unsalted butter

1 cup (250 mL) buttermilk
(or milk-vinegar substitute)

1 large egg

⅓ cup (75 mL) pure maple syrup

¾ cup (175 mL) crisp-cooked
bacon crumbles

¾ cup (175 mL) toffee bits

1 tsp (5 mL) cracked black pepper

Lightly spray with cooking oil or grease one or two large baking sheets. Line the baking sheets with parchment paper. Preheat the oven to 375°F (190°C).

Whisk together the tapioca starch, oat and sorghum flours, baking powder and salt in a medium bowl. Cut the butter into the mixture using two knives or a pastry cutter until it resembles coarse crumbs. Set aside. In a separate medium bowl, whisk the buttermilk, egg and maple syrup with the bacon and toffee bits. Gradually add the buttermilk mixture to the dry mixture in two or three batches, stirring until just moistened. Using a 1 Tbsp (15 mL) measure, scoop up the batter and gently shape it into balls. Place them on the prepared baking sheet 2 inches (5 cm) apart. Sprinkle the top of each scone with a pinch of fresh cracked black pepper. Flour your fingers and pat each scone gently to flatten. Bake for 16 to 18 minutes, until the edges are just beginning to turn lightly golden.

Allow to cool on the baking sheet and then either move them to a wire rack to cool completely or serve warm, right off the sheet.

PER SERVING: Energy 80 calories; Protein 1 g; Carbohydrates 10 g; Dietary Fiber 1 g; Fat 4 g; Sugar 2 g; Cholesterol 15 mg; Sodium 60 mg

STORAGE

Room Temperature: airtight container or bag, 2 days

Refrigerator: airtight container or bag, 2 days

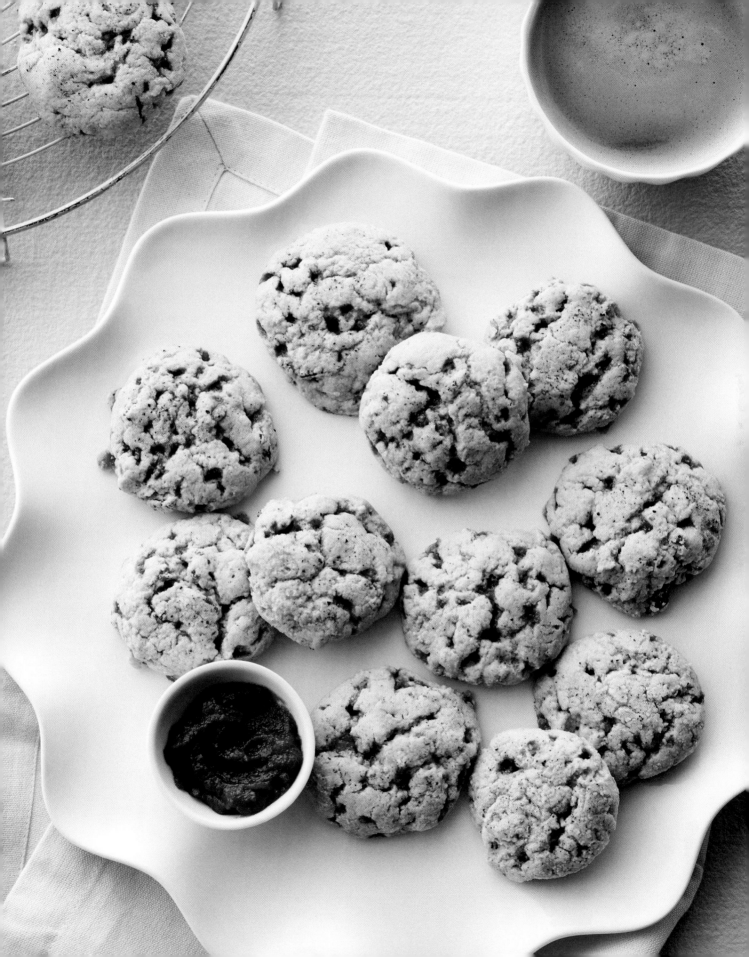

Cranberry, Walnut and Rosemary Muffins

This simple, lightly sweetened muffin with a blend of sorghum, millet and oat flours has a gentle hint of rosemary that deepens the flavor without making it savory.

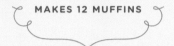

MAKES 12 MUFFINS

1 Tbsp (15 mL) ground chia seeds

¼ cup (60 mL) boiling water

⅔ cup (150 mL) sorghum flour

⅔ cup (150 mL) millet flour

⅔ cup (150 mL) oat flour

1 tsp (5 mL) baking soda

¼ tsp (1 mL) salt

½ cup (125 mL) organic
cane sugar

⅓ cup (75 mL) unsalted butter,
softened

1 large egg

1 cup (250 mL) 0% plain yogurt

1 cup (250 mL) unsweetened
applesauce

½ cup (125 mL) chopped,
sweetened dried cranberries

⅓ cup (75 mL) chopped walnuts

½ tsp (2 mL) finely chopped
fresh rosemary

Place paper muffin cup liners in a 12-cup muffin pan. Preheat the oven to 400°F (200°C).

Add the chia to the boiling water in a small bowl. Gently stir with a fork to ensure the ground seeds are evenly distributed. Set aside to thicken, about 10 minutes.

Place the sorghum, millet and oat flours, baking soda and salt in a large bowl and mix well. Set aside.

In a medium bowl, beat the sugar and butter, then mix in the chia mixture, egg, yogurt and applesauce. Add the applesauce mixture to the flour mixture and stir until just blended. Add the cranberries, walnuts and rosemary. Using a scoop or ladle, evenly distribute the batter among the muffin cups.

Bake for 22 to 24 minutes, until the muffin tops are slightly golden, the tops bounce back when pressed and a toothpick inserted in the center comes out with only a few crumbs. Remove from the oven and let sit in the muffin pan until cool.

PER SERVING: Energy 210 calories; Protein 5 g; Carbohydrates 30 g; Dietary Fiber 3 g; Fat 9 g; Sugar 15 g; Cholesterol 30 mg; Sodium 170 mg

STORAGE

Room Temperature: airtight container or bag, 5 days

Refrigerator: airtight container or bag, 5 days

Freezer: airtight freezer bag or container, 2 weeks

Strawberry Jam Oat Muffins

Completely butter- and oil-free, these moist and fluffy oat
and sorghum muffins have a sweet strawberry center.

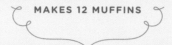

MAKES 12 MUFFINS

Place paper muffin cup liners in a 12-cup muffin pan. Preheat the oven to 375°F (190°C).

Place the oat and sorghum flours, tapioca starch, baking powder, salt and cinnamon in a large bowl and mix to combine. Add the oats and brown sugar and mix to combine. Set aside.

In a separate medium bowl, mix together the buttermilk and yogurt. Add the egg and vanilla and mix well. Add the buttermilk mixture to the flour mixture and stir until just blended. Using a scoop or ladle, fill the muffin cups halfway (you should still have a bit of batter remaining; reserve it). Add approximately ½ tsp (2 mL) of strawberry jam on top of each cup of batter. Top up each muffin cup, distributing the remaining batter evenly.

Bake for 14 to 16 minutes, until the muffin tops are lightly golden and a toothpick inserted in the center comes out with only a few crumbs. Remove from the oven and let cool in the muffin pan.

PER SERVING: Energy 100 calories; Protein 4 g; Carbohydrates 19 g; Dietary Fiber 2 g; Fat 1.5 g; Sugar 5 g; Cholesterol 15 mg; Sodium 130 mg

⅓ cup (75 mL) oat flour

⅓ cup (75 mL) sorghum flour

⅓ cup (75 mL) tapioca starch

2 tsp (10 mL) baking powder

½ tsp (2 mL) salt

¼ tsp (1 mL) cinnamon

1 cup (250 mL) quick oats

⅓ cup (75 mL) lightly packed brown sugar

1 cup (250 mL) buttermilk (or milk-vinegar substitute)

¼ cup (60 mL) 0% plain Greek yogurt

1 large egg

1 tsp (5 mL) pure vanilla extract

2 Tbsp (30 mL) strawberry jam or preserves

STORAGE

Room Temperature: airtight container or bag, 5 days

Refrigerator: airtight container or bag, 5 days

Freezer: airtight freezer bag or container, 2 weeks

Sweet Potato Muffins

Sweet potato is not only a great source of beta-carotene but also a good source of dietary fiber, iron and potassium. Combined with the goodness of sorghum flour, these dense but moist muffins are bursting with fall spices and flavor.

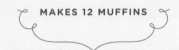

MAKES 12 MUFFINS

MUFFINS

1 cup (250 mL) sorghum flour

¾ cup (175 mL) white rice flour

1 ½ tsp (7 mL) baking powder

½ tsp (2 mL) baking soda

1 tsp (5 mL) cinnamon

½ tsp (2 mL) ground ginger

¼ tsp (1 mL) ground cloves

¼ tsp (1 mL) salt

⅔ cup (150 mL) seedless raisins

1 cup (250 mL) sweet potato,
    cooked in skin and flesh
    removed and mashed

2 large eggs

½ cup (125 mL) 2% milk
    or light coconut milk

⅓ cup (75 mL) liquid honey

⅓ cup (75 mL) grapeseed oil

1 Tbsp (15 mL) molasses

TOPPING

2 Tbsp (30 mL) shelled, raw
    unsalted pumpkin seeds
    (pepitas) or 1 Tbsp (15 mL)
    shelled, raw unsalted pumpkin
    seeds (pepitas) and 1 Tbsp
    (15 mL) raw, chopped walnuts

2 tsp (10 mL) liquid honey
    or pure maple syrup

Lightly spray with cooking oil, grease or line with paper muffin cup liners a 12-cup muffin tin. Preheat the oven to 375°F (190°C).

For the muffins, whisk together the sorghum and rice flours, baking powder, baking soda, cinnamon, ginger, cloves and salt in a medium bowl. Stir in the raisins and set aside.

Place the sweet potato flesh, eggs, milk, honey, oil and molasses in a large bowl and beat to combine. Gradually add in the flour mixture and stir until fully combined. Divide the batter evenly among the 12 muffin cups.

For the topping, toss the pumpkin seeds and walnuts (if using) with the honey in a separate, small bowl. Divide among the tops of the muffin batter.

Bake for 18 to 20 minutes, or until a toothpick inserted in the center comes out clean. Remove from the oven and let cool in the muffin pan.

PER SERVING: Energy 240 calories; Protein 4 g; Carbohydrates 39 g; Dietary Fiber 3 g; Fat 8 g; Sugar 17 g; Cholesterol 30 mg; Sodium 130 mg

STORAGE
Refrigerator: airtight container or bag, 5 days
Freezer: airtight freezer bag or container, 1 month

Wild Blueberry
Buttermilk Bran Muffins

A long-time favorite, bran muffins have traditionally been made from wheat bran and wheat flour. These freezer-friendly muffins have been carefully recreated using sorghum flour, rice flour and psyllium to make a great-tasting gluten-free version bursting with blueberries. Wild blueberries are smaller but you can use conventional blueberries.

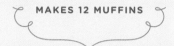

MAKES 12 MUFFINS

Lightly spray with cooking oil, grease or line with paper muffin cup liners a 12-cup muffin tin. Preheat the oven to 425°F (220°C).

Place the brown sugar, oil and molasses in a medium bowl and whisk until evenly mixed. Beat in the eggs, then add the buttermilk and then the bran.

In a separate large bowl, whisk together the sorghum and rice flours, psyllium, baking powder, baking soda and salt. Toss in the blueberries to coat them with flour. Stir in the sugar-oil mixture, stirring until just combined. Divide the batter evenly among the muffin cups.

Bake for 18 to 20 minutes, or until a toothpick inserted in the center comes out clean. Remove from the oven and let cool in the muffin pan.

PER SERVING: Energy 190 calories; Protein 5 g; Carbohydrates 32 g; Dietary Fiber 3 g; Fat 7 g; Sugar 14 g; Cholesterol 35 mg; Sodium 210 mg

½ cup (125 mL) lightly packed brown sugar

¼ cup (60 mL) grapeseed or organic light-tasting oil

¼ cup (60 mL) fancy molasses

2 large eggs

1¼ cups (310 mL) buttermilk (or milk-vinegar substitute)

1 cup (250 mL) oat bran

½ cup (125 mL) sorghum flour

½ cup (125 mL) sweet rice flour

1 tsp (5 mL) psyllium husks

1½ tsp (7 mL) baking powder

1 tsp (5 mL) baking soda

½ tsp (2 mL) salt

1⅓ cups (325 mL) fresh, wild or conventional blueberries

STORAGE

Refrigerator: **airtight container or bag, 4 days**

Freezer: **airtight freezer bag or container, 1 month**

BAKING TIP
Frozen berries can be used if they are thawed first. Thaw them in a single layer on a plate or baking sheet for about 30 minutes, prior to adding to the flour. Using berries that are too cold will prevent even baking in the muffins.

Nut and Chocolate Muffins

A soft, super-moist muffin made with oat, sorghum and quinoa flours.
Loaded with nutty flavor and topped with crunchy nuts, these muffins are unique.
Even made without the chocolate, they are scrumptious and are sure to disappear fast.

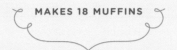

MAKES 18 MUFFINS

⅔ cup (150 mL) sorghum flour

⅔ cup (150 mL) oat flour

⅔ cup (150 mL) quinoa flour

½ cup (125 mL) tapioca starch

1 tsp (5 mL) baking soda

½ tsp (2 mL) salt

1 cup (250 mL) lightly packed
brown sugar

1 cup (250 mL) buttermilk
(or milk-vinegar substitute)

⅔ cup (150 mL) natural almond,
peanut or cashew butter
(smooth or crunchy)

¼ cup (60 mL) unsalted butter,
softened

2 large eggs

1 tsp (5 mL) pure vanilla extract

¼ cup (60 mL) milk chocolate
chunks

¼ cup (60 mL) chopped unsalted
almonds, peanuts or cashews
(optional)

Place paper muffin cup liners in three 6-cup muffin pans.
(If you only have 12-cup pans, use 18 cups and pour some
water into the other 6 to avoid burning them.) Preheat the
oven to 375°F (190°C).

Place the sorghum, oat and quinoa flours, tapioca starch,
baking soda and salt in a large bowl and mix to combine.
Mix in the brown sugar. Set aside.

In a separate medium bowl, mix the buttermilk, nut butter,
unsalted butter, eggs and vanilla together. Add the nut butter
mixture to the flour mixture and stir until just blended. Using
a scoop or ladle, fill the muffin cups halfway (you should still
have a bit of batter remaining; reserve it). Place a chocolate
chunk or two on top of each cup of batter. Top up each muffin
cup, distributing the remaining batter evenly. Sprinkle the tops
with chopped nuts (if using).

Bake for 17 to 19 minutes, until the muffin tops are slightly
golden and bounce back when pressed and a toothpick inserted
in the center comes out clean. Remove from the oven and let
cool in the pans.

PER SERVING: Energy 240 calories; Protein 6 g; Carbohydrates 28 g;
Dietary Fiber 3 g; Fat 12 g; Sugar 13 g; Cholesterol 35 mg; Sodium 190 mg

STORAGE
Refrigerator: airtight container or bag, 1 week
Freezer: airtight freezer bag or container, 2 weeks

Almond Ancient Grain Cupcakes

Sorghum, oat and quinoa flours add ancient grain goodness to these cakes that are loaded with almond flavor and topped with almond cream cheese frosting and toasted almonds.

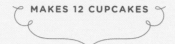

MAKES 12 CUPCAKES

Place paper muffin cup liners in a 12-cup muffin pan. Preheat the oven to 350°F (180°C).

For the cupcakes, place the sliced almonds on a baking sheet and bake for 5 to 7 minutes, until fragrant and toasted. Watch them closely, as they can burn quickly. Remove from the oven and let cool completely on the baking sheet.

Place the sorghum, oat and quinoa flours, tapioca starch, baking powder, baking soda and salt in a large bowl and mix to combine. Set aside.

In a separate medium bowl, mix the brown sugar with the buttermilk, yogurt, eggs, oil and almond and vanilla extracts to combine. Add the buttermilk mixture to the flour mixture and stir until just blended. Gently fold ¼ cup (60 mL) of the toasted almonds into the batter. Evenly distribute the batter among the 12 muffin cups.

Bake for 15 to 16 minutes, until the cake tops are lightly golden and spring back when pressed, and a toothpick inserted in the center comes out clean. Remove from the oven and allow to cool in the pan.

For the frosting, use a handheld mixer or rotary beater to mix together the powdered sugar, cream cheese, milk and the 1 ½ tsp (7 mL) almond extract until fluffy.

Frost the cupcakes, scattering the remaining toasted almonds on top.

PER SERVING (with frosting): Energy 260 calories; Protein 6 g; Carbohydrates 48 g; Dietary Fiber 2 g; Fat 4.5 g; Sugar 37 g; Cholesterol 35 mg; Sodium 220 mg

CUPCAKES

½ cup (125 mL) sliced almonds

⅓ cup (75 mL) sorghum or millet flour

⅓ cup (75 mL) oat flour

⅓ cup (75 mL) quinoa flour

⅓ cup (75 mL) tapioca starch

1 tsp (5 mL) baking powder

½ tsp (2 mL) baking soda

¼ tsp (1 mL) salt

½ cup (125 mL) lightly packed brown sugar

½ cup (125 mL) buttermilk (or milk-vinegar substitute)

¼ cup (60 mL) 1% plain yogurt

2 large eggs

1 Tbsp (15 mL) grapeseed or organic light-tasting oil

1 tsp (5 mL) pure almond extract

1 tsp (5 mL) pure vanilla extract

FROSTING

3 ½ cups (875 mL) powdered (icing) sugar

½ cup (125 mL) cream cheese, softened

¼ cup (60 mL) 1% or 2% milk or almond milk

1 ½ tsp (7 mL) pure almond extract

STORAGE
Room Temperature: **airtight container or bag, 1 week**

Honey Ginger Carrot Cakes with Lime Cream Cheese Frosting

Elevate the flavor of standard carrot cake with fresh ginger and honey. Frost these cakes with lime cream cheese frosting or your favorite frosting or glaze. Use a pan that makes individual brownies or a standard muffin tin if desired. Cut these beauties in half if you want to frost the middle too.

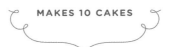

MAKES 10 CAKES

CAKES

¹⁄₃ cup (75 mL) millet
    or light buckwheat flour

¹⁄₃ cup (75 mL) coconut flour

¹⁄₃ cup (75 mL) oat flour

1 Tbsp (15 mL) psyllium husks

1 tsp (5 mL) baking powder

¹⁄₄ tsp (1 mL) baking soda

¹⁄₂ tsp (2 mL) cinnamon

¹⁄₂ tsp (2 mL) salt

2 large eggs

¹⁄₂ cup (125 mL) liquid honey

¹⁄₃ cup (75 mL) grapeseed
    or organic light-tasting oil

¹⁄₄ cup (60 mL) ground Sucanat
    or organic cane sugar

1 Tbsp + 1 tsp (20 mL) peeled
    and finely grated fresh ginger

1 ¹⁄₂ cups (375 mL) peeled and
    grated carrots

LIME CREAM CHEESE FROSTING

8 oz (250 g) package of light
    cream cheese, at room
    temperature

²⁄₃ cup (150 mL) thick Greek
    2% yogurt (or yogurt cheese
    from Mini Maple Cherry
    Cheesecakes, page 79)

2–3 Tbsp (30–45 mL) liquid honey

1 cup (250 mL) powdered
    (icing) sugar

1 Tbsp (15 mL) lime or lemon zest

1 tsp (5 mL) pure vanilla extract

Lightly grease or spray with cooking oil 10 cups in an individual brownie pan or a 12-cup muffin tin. Add water to the empty cups to prevent burning. Preheat the oven to 350°F (180°C).

For the cakes, place the millet, coconut and oat flours, psyllium, baking powder, baking soda, cinnamon and salt in a large bowl and whisk to combine. In a separate small bowl, whisk together the eggs, honey, grapeseed oil, sugar and ginger. Stir the grated carrot into the egg mixture. Stir the carrot-egg mixture into the flour mixture until fully incorporated. Fill ten of the brownie or muffin tins halfway.

Bake for 18 to 20 minutes, or until a toothpick inserted in the center comes out clean and the edges of the cakes are golden. Let cool completely in the pan.

For the frosting, beat the cream cheese in a stand mixer or in a bowl with a handheld mixer until smooth. Add the yogurt and honey gradually, while the machine is running on low, until incorporated. Stir in the zest and vanilla and mix well. Decorate the cakes as desired, using about 2 Tbsp (30 mL) of frosting per cake. Any leftover frosting can be kept refrigerated in an airtight container for up to a week.

PER SERVING: Energy 280 calories; Protein 6 g; Carbohydrates 38 g; Dietary Fiber 4 g; Fat 11 g; Sugar 24 g; Cholesterol 50 mg; Sodium 190 mg

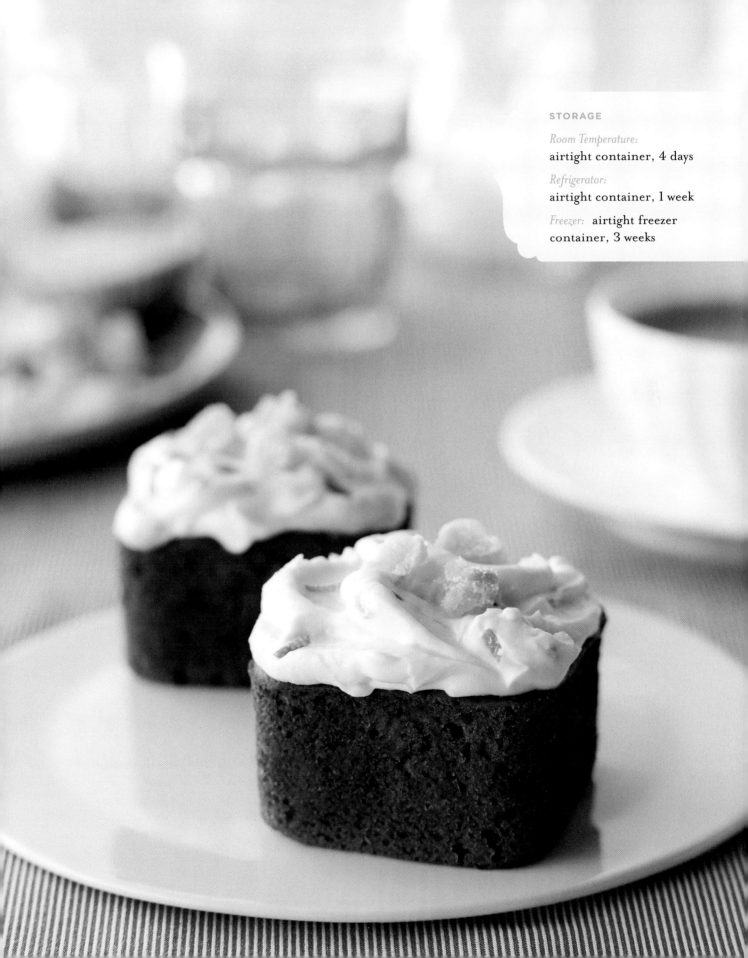

STORAGE

Room Temperature:
airtight container, 4 days

Refrigerator:
airtight container, 1 week

Freezer: airtight freezer
container, 3 weeks

BAKING TIP
Avoid a mess by placing a resealable plastic bag in a shallow glass. Use a spatula to put all the batter into the bag. Seal the bag and cut ¾ inch (2 cm) off one corner. Pipe the batter into the doughnut tin.

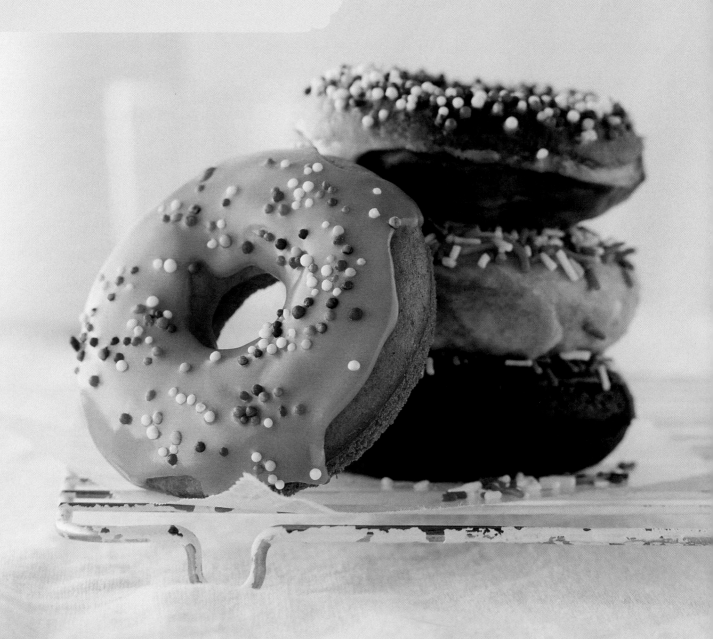

Old-Fashioned Cake Doughnuts

Old-Fashioned Cake Doughnuts are a nostalgic treat. Baked instead of deep-fried, they are a much more modern and certainly healthier option. Allow yourself to enjoy them occasionally by baking them in a doughnut pan. If you don't have one, use a mini muffin tin instead, but keep a watchful eye on them while they are in the oven so they don't overbake. You can easily double this recipe if desired.

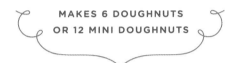

**MAKES 6 DOUGHNUTS
OR 12 MINI DOUGHNUTS**

Lightly spray with cooking oil or grease a doughnut baking pan (or mini muffin tin). Preheat the oven to 375°F (190°C).

Place the sorghum flour, tapioca starch, oat flour, psyllium, baking powder, nutmeg, xanthan gum and salt in a medium bowl and whisk to combine. Set aside.

In a separate small bowl, lightly whisk the egg and honey. Add the milk, butter and vanilla, whisking until well combined. Pour the milk mixture into the flour mixture and stir until thoroughly combined. Pour the batter halfway up each doughnut mold (or mini muffin cup).

Bake for 10 minutes, or until the bottoms are lightly golden and a toothpick inserted in the center comes out clean. Let cool completely in the pan, then remove and decorate as desired. Dust with powdered (icing) sugar for a quick finish. (See page 13 if you want to make your own powdered sugar.)

PER SERVING: Energy 150 calories; Protein 3 g; Carbohydrates 26 g; Dietary Fiber 3 g; Fat 4.5 g; Sugar 9 g; Cholesterol 40 mg; Sodium 70 mg

½ cup (125 mL) sorghum flour

¼ cup (60 mL) tapioca starch

2 Tbsp (30 mL) oat flour

1 tsp (5 mL) psyllium husks

¾ tsp (3 mL) baking powder

½ tsp (2 mL) nutmeg

¼ tsp (1 mL) xanthan gum

pinch salt

1 large egg

¼ cup (60 mL) liquid honey

3 Tbsp (45 mL) 1% milk
  or milk substitute

3 Tbsp (45 mL) melted unsalted
  butter or virgin coconut oil

½ tsp (2 mL) pure vanilla extract

STORAGE

Room Temperature: **airtight container or bag, 1 day**

Double Chocolate Cake Doughnuts

Decorate them as fancy as you wish! Light yet not shy on double chocolaty flavor and made with sorghum and teff flour, these doughnuts don't have to be fried to be good.

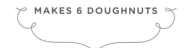

MAKES 6 DOUGHNUTS

DOUGHNUTS

⅓ cup (75 mL) sorghum flour

⅓ cup (75 mL) teff flour

¼ cup (60 mL) unsweetened cocoa powder

1 tsp (5 mL) baking powder

¼ tsp (1 mL) salt

¼ tsp (1 mL) xanthan gum

1 large egg

⅓ cup (75 mL) liquid honey

3 Tbsp (45 mL) unsalted butter, melted, or virgin coconut oil

¼ cup (60 mL) 1% milk or milk substitute

GLAZE

1 cup (250 mL) powdered (icing) sugar

3 Tbsp (45 mL) unsweetened cocoa powder

1 tsp (5 mL) pure vanilla extract

Sprinkles, nuts or toasted coconut for decorating (optional)

Lightly spray with cooking oil or grease a doughnut baking pan. Preheat the oven to 375°F (190°C).

For the doughnuts, place the sorghum and teff flours, cocoa, baking powder, salt and xanthan gum in a medium bowl and whisk to combine. Set aside.

In a separate large bowl, whisk the egg, honey and butter. Add the milk and whisk until incorporated. Gradually stir in the flour mixture until thoroughly mixed. Pour the batter three-quarters of the way up each doughnut mold. Bake for 12 to 15 minutes, or until a toothpick inserted in the center comes out clean. Transfer to a rack to cool completely.

Place the cooling rack of doughnuts on a large baking sheet and set aside while you make the glaze.

For the glaze, gently stir together the sugar and cocoa in a medium bowl. Slowly add in the vanilla and then 2 to 3 tsp (10–15 mL) of water, a little at a time, until you have a smooth glaze. Dip one side of a doughnut in the glaze and place on the cooling rack to allow the excess glaze to drip off. While the glaze is wet, decorate with sprinkles, nuts or coconut (if using). Allow the glaze to set for 30 minutes before serving.

PER SERVING: Energy 230 calories; Protein 5 g; Carbohydrates 36 g; Dietary Fiber 4 g; Fat 8 g; Sugar 21 g; Cholesterol 45 mg; Sodium 105 mg

STORAGE

Room Temperature: **slightly open container, 1 day**

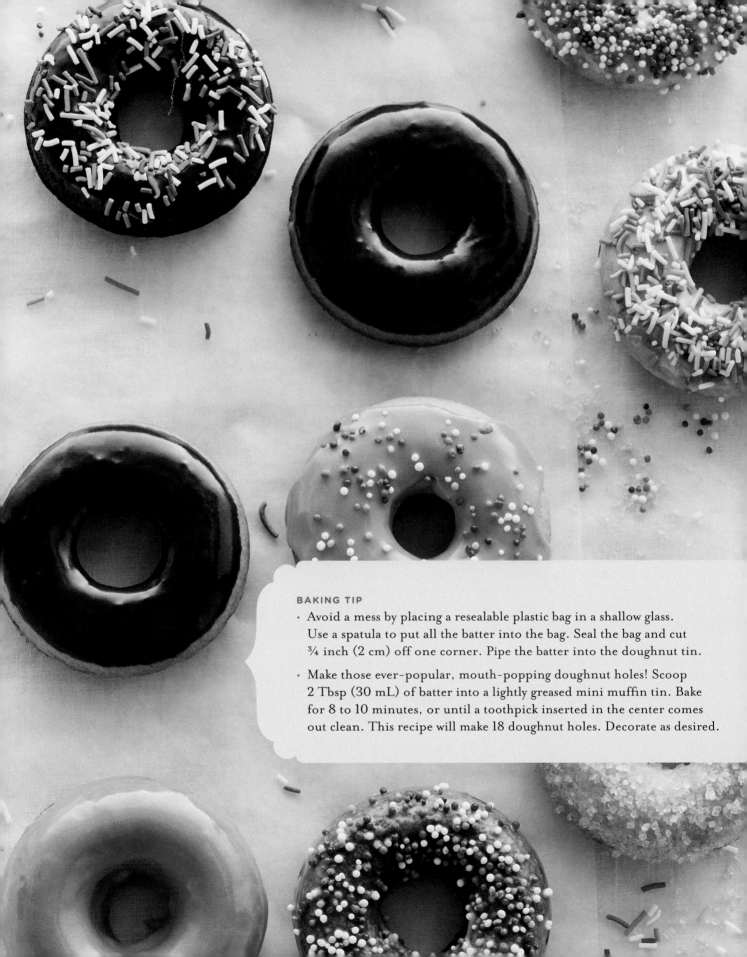

BAKING TIP

- Avoid a mess by placing a resealable plastic bag in a shallow glass. Use a spatula to put all the batter into the bag. Seal the bag and cut ¾ inch (2 cm) off one corner. Pipe the batter into the doughnut tin.

- Make those ever-popular, mouth-popping doughnut holes! Scoop 2 Tbsp (30 mL) of batter into a lightly greased mini muffin tin. Bake for 8 to 10 minutes, or until a toothpick inserted in the center comes out clean. This recipe will make 18 doughnut holes. Decorate as desired.

Banana Breakfast Bread

Begin the day with a moist piece of banana bread loaded with nutritious ingredients such as sorghum, oats, dates, walnuts and cranberries. Play with the types of dried fruit and nuts you have on hand. Pair it with some yogurt and fresh fruit for a well-balanced breakfast.

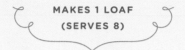

**MAKES 1 LOAF
(SERVES 8)**

⅓ cup (75 mL) sorghum flour

⅓ cup (75 mL) oat flour

⅓ cup (75 mL) quinoa
or light buckwheat flour

1 tsp (5 mL) baking soda

¼ tsp (1 mL) salt

¼ cup (60 mL) finely chopped
Medjool dates

¼ cup (60 mL) finely chopped
walnuts or pecans

¼ cup (60 mL) sweetened dried
cranberries

2 large eggs

⅓ cup (75 mL) unsweetened
applesauce

¼ cup (60 mL) grapeseed
or organic light-tasting oil

⅓ cup (75 mL) lightly packed
brown sugar

1 cup (250 mL) mashed ripe
banana

Lightly grease a 9- × 5-inch (2 L) loaf pan. Line the sides and the bottom with one piece of parchment paper and lightly grease the parchment. Preheat the oven to 350°F (180°C).

Whisk together the sorghum, oat and quinoa flours, baking soda and salt in a small bowl. Stir in the dates, walnuts and cranberries, using your hands to separate the cranberries, if necessary. Set aside.

In a separate medium bowl, mix together the eggs, applesauce, oil, brown sugar and banana. Stir the dry ingredients into the wet until just mixed. Pour the batter into the prepared loaf pan.

Bake for 40 to 45 minutes, or until a toothpick inserted in the center comes out clean. Cool slightly in the pan, then transfer to a wire rack. Slice while still warm or wait until it has cooled completely.

PER SERVING: Energy 230 calories; Protein 4 g; Carbohydrates 31 g; Dietary Fiber 3 g; Fat 11 g; Sugar 16 g; Cholesterol 45 mg; Sodium 190 mg

STORAGE
Refrigerator: airtight bag, 4 days
Freezer: airtight freezer bag, 2 weeks

Breakfast Popover Loaf

This fluffy and chewy popover loaf is similar in texture to Yorkshire pudding. It makes a great light dish all on its own or as a brunch option next to just about anything you want to serve for breakfast. The flavor can be sweet or savory and completely customized depending on your taste. Try any of the flavor combinations suggested in our baking tip, or experiment with your own.

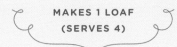

**MAKES 1 LOAF
(SERVES 4)**

Preheat the oven to 450°F (230°C). Generously spray with cooking oil or grease an 8 ½- × 4 ½-inch (1.5 L) loaf pan and place it in the preheating oven to warm.

Place the oat and quinoa flours, tapioca starch and salt in a medium bowl and mix to combine. Set aside.

In a separate medium bowl, beat the eggs and milk. Add the melted butter and vanilla and continue to beat. Stir into the flour mixture to combine.

Remove the pan from the oven. Pour the batter into the loaf pan and bake for 15 minutes. Turn down the oven heat to 400°F (200°C) and bake for another 22 to 25 minutes, until the top is puffed and golden. Serve immediately. The loaf will fall as soon as you cut into it. Serve each slice with a drizzle of maple syrup and fresh berries (if using).

Best eaten the day you make it.

PER SERVING: Energy 260 calories; Protein 11 g; Carbohydrates 27 g; Dietary Fiber 3 g; Fat 11 g; Sugar 4 g; Cholesterol 140 mg; Sodium 210 mg

½ cup (125 mL) oat flour

½ cup (125 mL) quinoa flour

¼ cup (60 mL) tapioca starch

¼ tsp (1 mL) salt

3 large eggs

1 ¼ cups (310 mL) 1% or 2% milk

2 Tbsp (30 ml) melted unsalted butter

1 tsp (5 mL) pure vanilla extract

¼ cup (60 mL) maple syrup (optional)

1 cup (250 mL) assorted fresh berries (optional)

BAKING TIP
Instead of fruit and maple syrup, try adding a pinch of cayenne, aged Cheddar cheese and chopped jalapeños or fresh fruit, cinnamon sugar, apple butter, or fresh preserves or simply a light dusting of powdered sugar.

Prune Spice Loaf

Buckwheat and ground cloves make for a delicious combination in this tasty loaf sweetened with prunes. Sorghum, oats, coconut oil and cinnamon round out the flavor profile nicely.

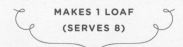

**MAKES 1 LOAF
(SERVES 8)**

1 cup (250 mL) light buckwheat flour

½ cup (125 mL) oat flour

½ cup (125 mL) sorghum flour

¼ cup (60 mL) tapioca starch

1 tsp (5 mL) baking powder

1 tsp (5 mL) baking soda

2 tsp (10 mL) cinnamon

½ tsp (2 mL) ground cloves

½ tsp (2 mL) salt

½ cup (125 mL) lightly packed brown sugar

⅓ cup (75 mL) virgin coconut oil

2 large eggs

1 cup (250 mL) unsweetened applesauce

⅓ cup (75 mL) 1% plain yogurt

1 tsp (5 mL) pure vanilla extract

¾ cup (175 mL) chopped, dried prunes

Lightly grease or spray with cooking oil a 9- × 5-inch (2 L) loaf pan. Line the pan with parchment paper. Preheat the oven to 350°F (180°C).

Place the buckwheat, oat and sorghum flours, tapioca starch, baking powder, baking soda, cinnamon, cloves and salt in a medium bowl and whisk to combine. Set aside.

In a separate medium bowl, beat the brown sugar and coconut oil. Add the eggs, applesauce, yogurt and vanilla and mix thoroughly. Add the prunes. Stir the wet mixture into the flour mixture until well combined. Pour the batter into the prepared pan.

Bake for 45 to 50 minutes, until a toothpick inserted in the center comes out with only a few crumbs. Do not overbake. Let the loaf cool slightly in the pan before moving it to a wire rack. Slice while still warm or wait until it has cooled completely.

PER SERVING: Energy 260 calories; Protein 6 g; Carbohydrates 37 g; Dietary Fiber 5 g; Fat 9 g; Sugar 17 g; Cholesterol 45 mg; Sodium 130 mg

BAKING TIP
Using room-temperature eggs helps with the "lift" in quick bread recipes and also helps to bind and make a better crumb.

STORAGE
Refrigerator: airtight container, 1 week

Chocolate Swirl Banana Loaf

This nutritious loaf is made with the wholesomeness of sorghum, millet and oat flours, bananas and applesauce. It is sweetened with brown sugar and a delicious swirl of chocolate.

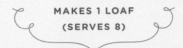

**MAKES 1 LOAF
(SERVES 8)**

Lightly grease or spray with cooking oil a 9- × 5-inch (2 L) loaf pan. Line the pan with parchment paper. Preheat the oven to 350°F (180°C).

Place the oat, millet and sorghum flours, baking soda and salt in a medium bowl and whisk to combine. Set aside.

In a separate medium bowl, whisk together the egg, egg whites, banana, brown sugar, applesauce and oil. Gently stir the egg mixture into the flour mixture until just mixed. Pour half of the batter into the prepared loaf pan and set the remainder aside for a moment.

Melt the chocolate chips in a double boiler over low heat until just melted. Pour the melted chocolate on top of the batter in the loaf pan. Top with the remaining batter and run a knife through the mixture to swirl the chocolate. Repeat a few times until the desired swirl is achieved.

Bake for 40 to 45 minutes, until a toothpick inserted in the center comes out clean. Let the loaf cool slightly in the pan before moving it to a wire rack. Slice while still warm or wait until it has cooled completely.

⅓ cup (75 mL) oat flour

⅓ cup (75 mL) millet flour

⅓ cup (75 mL) sorghum flour

1 tsp (5 mL) baking soda

¼ tsp (1 mL) salt

1 large egg

2 large egg whites

1 cup (250 mL) mashed ripe banana

⅓ cup (75 mL) lightly packed brown sugar

⅓ cup (75 mL) unsweetened applesauce

¼ tsp (1 mL) grapeseed or organic light-tasting oil

½ cup (125 mL) semisweet chocolate chips

PER SERVING: Energy 160 calories; Protein 4 g; Carbohydrates 27 g; Dietary Fiber 3 g; Fat 4.5 g; Sugar 15 g; Cholesterol 25 mg; Sodium 260 mg

STORAGE

Refrigerator: airtight container or bag, 1 week

Maple Raisin Cinnamon Buns

Tender cinnamon buns with raisins and a gooey sauce fresh out of the oven are a serious treat. Make them for coffee with friends, for brunch or just for fun. These are fabulous reheated the next day. (Note that you can't use quick-rising yeast for these.)

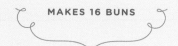

MAKES 16 BUNS

SAUCE

¼ cup (60 mL) lightly packed brown sugar

¼ cup (60 mL) pure maple syrup or liquid honey

¼ cup (60 mL) unsalted butter

1 Tbsp (15 mL) 1% milk or milk substitute

2 tsp (10 mL) pure vanilla extract

DOUGH

1 ¼ cups (310 mL) warm 1% milk or milk substitute at 100–105°F (40–41°C)

1 Tbsp (15 mL) organic cane sugar

2 Tbsp (30 mL) dry active yeast (NOT quick-rising)

¼ cup (60 mL) unsalted butter, melted

⅓ cup (75 mL) organic cane sugar

2 large eggs

2 tsp (10 mL) pure vanilla extract

1 cup (250 mL) sweet rice flour

¾ cup (175 mL) sorghum flour

¾ cup (175 mL) potato starch

¾ cup (175 mL) tapioca starch

1 ½ tsp (7 mL) xanthan gum

½ tsp (2 mL) salt

1 tsp (5 mL) baking powder

½ tsp (2 mL) cream of tartar

FILLING

⅓ cup (75 mL) unsalted butter, very soft

¾ cup (175 mL) lightly packed brown sugar

1 ½ tsp (7 mL) cinnamon

½ cup (125 mL) seedless raisins, plump or hydrated

STORAGE

Room Temperature: airtight container or bag, 3 days

Refrigerator: airtight container or bag, 4 days

Lightly grease a 13- × 9-inch (3.5 L) baking dish.

For the sauce, warm the brown sugar, maple syrup and butter in a small saucepan until the butter has melted. Stir in the milk and vanilla. Pour this into the bottom of the baking dish and spread it evenly across the bottom.

For the dough, mix the warm milk with the sugar in a medium bowl and sprinkle the yeast overtop of the milk. Stir the yeast slightly so it is still floating but is evenly touching the milk surface. Cover and place in a warm, draft-free area to activate for 8 to 10 minutes (most of the yeast should be activated). The yeast will look like a creamy foam.

In a separate medium bowl, whisk the butter with the sugar, eggs and vanilla until combined. Once the yeast has been activated, whisk it into the butter-egg mixture until combined and set aside.

Whisk the sweet rice and sorghum flours, potato and tapioca starch, xanthan gum, salt, baking powder and cream of tartar in the bowl of a stand mixer. While the machine is running, slowly add the yeast mixture into the flour mixture. Mix on low speed with the paddle attachment until combined. The dough will be sticky. Mix for 2 additional minutes on medium speed.

Tape a piece of parchment paper at least 22 × 10 inches (55 × 25 cm) to a flat surface. Dust the parchment paper with sweet rice flour or tapioca starch, and flour your hands. Turn the sticky dough onto the parchment. Use your hands to pat the dough into a flattened rectangle, sprinkle the top with flour, then roll it into a rectangle 22 inches (55 cm) long and 10 inches (25 cm) wide. Periodically check that the dough is not sticking to the parchment. Sprinkle with more flour as needed.

For the filling, spread the top of the dough evenly with softened butter, being careful not to pull excessively on the dough (if the butter is not spreading, let it soften some more). Sprinkle the dough evenly with brown sugar, then cinnamon and raisins. Pulling on the parchment to help you, roll from the long side of the dough, ensuring it rolls tightly, until it becomes a log. Pinch the edge against the main body of the log. Score the dough into 16 pieces (each piece will be slightly wider than 1 inch/2.5 cm). Cut gently into rolls by using a sharp knife. Be careful not to flatten the slices.

Delicately place the rolls in the baking pan, spacing them evenly. Place them in a warm, draft-free area, covered with a dry towel, until doubled in size, 50 minutes to 1 hour.

Preheat the oven to 375°F (190°C).

Bake for 30 minutes, covering the pan with aluminum foil when the tops have become golden. (Start checking 15 minutes into the baking time.) Remove from the oven, discard the foil and let sit in the pan for 10 minutes before serving. Serve warm or cool.

BAKING TIP
If desired, drizzle with glaze (page 68).

PER SERVING: Energy 270 calories; Protein 3 g; Carbohydrates 42 g; Dietary Fiber 1 g; Fat 11 g; Sugar 20 g; Cholesterol 50 mg; Sodium 95 mg

Raspberry Lemon Quinoa and Oat Loaves

Sweet and lemony individual mini-sized loaves made with pureed cooked quinoa and oats. Use fresh lemon zest for the best flavor.

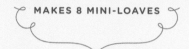

MAKES 8 MINI-LOAVES

¼ cup (60 mL) white or golden quinoa seeds

½ cup (125 mL) lightly packed brown sugar

1 cup (250 mL) unsweetened applesauce

2 Tbsp (30 mL) pure maple syrup

2 Tbsp (30 mL) grapeseed or organic light-tasting oil

1 large egg

2 tsp (10 mL) fresh lemon juice

2 tsp (10 mL) lemon zest

1 cup (250 mL) oat flour

1 ½ tsp (7 mL) baking powder

½ tsp (2 mL) salt

½ tsp (2 mL) cinnamon

1 ½ cups (375 mL) fresh or frozen (thawed, drained) raspberries

Lightly grease or spray with cooking oil one 8-cavity mini-loaf pan and line it with paper liners. Preheat the oven to 400°F (200°C).

Place the quinoa in a medium saucepan with ½ cup (125 mL) of water and bring to a boil. Cover the pan, turn down the heat to a simmer and cook for 10 minutes. Turn off the heat and leave the covered saucepan on the burner for another 15 minutes. Fluff the quinoa with a fork and allow to cool.

Place the quinoa in a food processor or blender and puree it with the brown sugar, applesauce, maple syrup, oil, egg, lemon juice and zest and set aside.

In a medium bowl, whisk together the flour, baking powder, salt and cinnamon. Gently toss the raspberries into the flour mixture. Add the pureed quinoa mixture to the flour mixture, stirring until just blended and being careful not to overmix. Divide the batter evenly among the loaf cups.

Bake for 35 to 37 minutes, or until a toothpick inserted in the center of a loaf comes out clean. Let cool in the pan.

PER SERVING: Energy 170 calories; Protein 3 g; Carbohydrates 29 g; Dietary Fiber 3 g; Fat 5 g; Sugar 15 g; Cholesterol 25 mg; Sodium 150 mg

BAKING TIP
If you don't have raspberries, try blueberries.

STORAGE
Refrigerator: airtight container, 4 days

Mint Chocolate-Dipped Cake Bites

This cake made of oat, millet and sorghum flours is enhanced with coconut oil, baked until soft and chewy and then cut into bite-sized cubes that are dipped in mint chocolate.

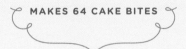

MAKES 64 CAKE BITES

Lightly grease or spray with cooking oil an 8-inch (2 L) square baking pan. Line the pan with parchment paper. Preheat the oven to 375°F (190°C).

For the cake, place the oat, millet and sorghum flours, baking powder and salt in a medium bowl and mix to combine. Set aside.

In a separate medium bowl, mix the oil with the sugar, then add the eggs, buttermilk and vanilla. Add the buttermilk mixture to the flour mixture and stir well. Pour the batter evenly into the prepared pan.

Bake for 28 to 30 minutes, until the top springs back when gently pressed or a toothpick inserted in the center comes out with only a few small crumbs. Set aside to cool in the pan.

For the frosting, place the powdered sugar and cocoa powder in a small bowl with the boiling water and mix well. Add the mint extract.

Line a large baking sheet with parchment paper.

Slice the cooled cake into 64 cubes. Dip each cube in chocolate and place it on the baking sheet. Refrigerate until the chocolate hardens.

PER SERVING (4–5 cake bites): Energy 160 calories; Protein 4 g; Carbohydrates 20 g; Dietary Fiber 2 g; Fat 6 g; Sugar 12 g; Cholesterol 20 mg; Sodium 200 mg

CAKE

²/₃ cup (150 mL) oat flour

¹/₃ cup (75 mL) millet flour

¹/₃ cup (75 mL) sorghum flour

1 Tbsp (15 mL) baking powder

¹/₂ tsp (2 mL) salt

¹/₂ cup (125 mL) virgin coconut oil

¹/₂ cup (125 mL) organic cane sugar

2 large eggs

1 cup (250 mL) buttermilk (or milk-vinegar substitute)

1 tsp (5 mL) pure vanilla extract

FROSTING

1 ¹/₂ cups (375 mL) powdered (icing) sugar

¹/₃ cup (75 mL) unsweetened cocoa powder

¹/₄–¹/₂ cup (60–125 mL) boiling water

¹/₂ tsp (2 mL) mint extract

STORAGE

Refrigerator: airtight container, 1 day

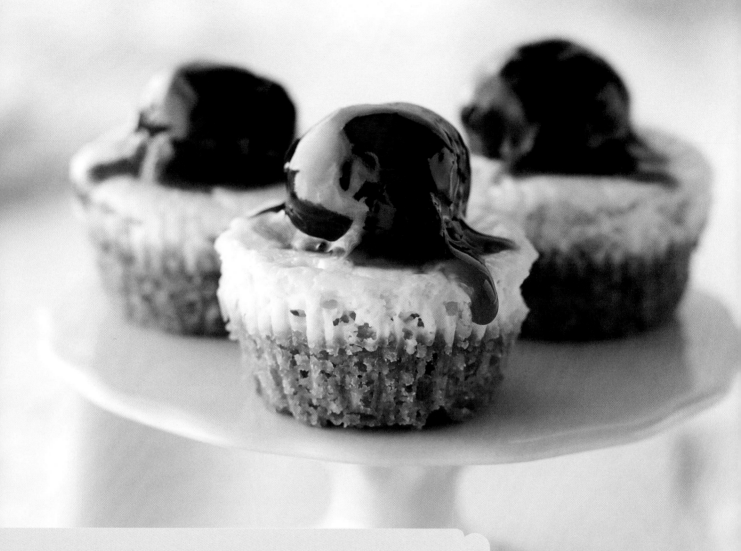

BAKING TIP

· Top with chocolate, blackberry or strawberry sauce, or any of your favorite cheesecake toppings.

· You must use yogurt with no gelatin. It will likely be clearly labeled if it does not contain gelatin, but if it is not obvious, do ensure that it is not on the product's list of ingredients. Yogurt that contains gelatin will not allow retained water to drain off.

· Make mini cheesecakes a larger handheld version by using regular-sized muffin pans. Use a ¼ cup/60 mL scoop of cheesecake mixture per cup and bake for the same amount of time as the mini version.

Mini Maple Cherry Cheesecakes

Just the perfect size, and with fewer calories than regular cheesecake! Use the Graham-Style Wafer Crumb Crust (page 108) to make individual cheesecakes with plain yogurt (yogurt cheese) instead of cream cheese. A beautiful, petite and delectable dessert that is lovely for serving to guests or simply for exercising portion control. Give yourself time, though — you need to let the yogurt sit overnight to thicken and drain!

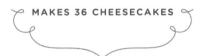 **MAKES 36 CHEESECAKES**

Line a large sieve with paper towels and place it on top of a medium bowl. Place the yogurt inside the strainer and allow to rest overnight in the refrigerator. The yogurt will drain and thicken. Prepare the crusts at this time as well so they're ready to use at the same time as the yogurt.

Preheat the oven to 325°F (160°C).

Discard the liquid from the yogurt and measure 2 cups (500 mL) of the firmed and thickened yogurt (yogurt cheese) into a large bowl. Add the eggs, maple syrup, 1 Tbsp (15 mL) of the cornstarch and vanilla. Using a rotary hand beater, handheld mixer or immersion blender, beat the mixture until well blended. Using a tablespoon, scoop the cheesecake mixture into the individual crusts. Bake for 13 to 15 minutes, until the cheesecakes are firm. Remove from the oven and allow to cool.

Meanwhile, in a medium saucepan over high heat, combine the cherries and their syrup with the remaining 2 tsp (10 mL) cornstarch and 1 cup (250 mL) of water. Bring to a boil. Turn down the heat to a simmer and stir constantly until the mixture thickens slightly, about 10 minutes. Remove from the heat and allow to cool completely.

When the cheesecakes and sauce have cooled, chill them in the refrigerator for 1 hour. Top each mini cheesecake with cherry syrup to serve.

PER SERVING: Energy 60 calories; Protein 2 g; Carbohydrates 9 g; Dietary Fiber 1 g; Fat 2 g; Sugar 6 g; Cholesterol 20 mg; Sodium 30 mg

3 ½ cups (875 mL) 1% or 2% plain yogurt (no gelatin)

36 prepared and baked mini Graham-Style Wafer Crumb Crusts (page 108)

3 large eggs, beaten

⅓ cup (75 mL) pure maple syrup

1 Tbsp + 2 tsp (25 mL) cornstarch

2 tsp (10 mL) pure vanilla extract

1 ½ cups (375 mL) or one 14 oz/398 mL can Bing cherries in light syrup

1 cup (250 mL) water

1 Tbsp (15 mL) pure maple syrup

STORAGE

Room Temperature:
airtight container, 1 day

Refrigerator:
airtight container, 4 days

Ancient Grain Pound Cake

An easy-to-make moist and sweet pound cake — made gluten-free with ancient grains.
Great on its own or versatile for use in any dessert that requires conventional pound cake.

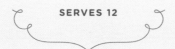

SERVES 12

¾ cup (175 mL) quinoa flour

½ cup (125 mL) oat flour

¼ cup (60 mL) tapioca starch

2 tsp (10 mL) baking powder

¼ tsp (1 mL) salt

½ cup (125 mL) unsalted butter

¾ cup (175 mL) organic
    cane sugar

3 large eggs

½ cup (125 mL) 0% plain yogurt

2 tsp (10 mL) pure vanilla extract

Preheat the oven to 350°F (180°C). Lightly spray with cooking oil or grease a 9- × 5-inch (2 L) loaf pan and place it in the preheating oven to warm.

Place the quinoa and oat flours, tapioca starch, baking powder and salt in a medium bowl and mix to combine. Set aside.

In a separate medium bowl, beat the butter with the sugar. Add the eggs, yogurt and vanilla and mix well. Stir in the flour mixture and mix until just combined. Remove the loaf pan from the oven and pour the batter into it.

Bake for 45 to 50 minutes, until a toothpick inserted in the center comes out with only a few small crumbs. Let cool completely in the pan.

PER SERVING: Energy 190 calories; Protein 4 g; Carbohydrates 23 g; Dietary Fiber 1 g; Fat 10 g; Sugar 13 g; Cholesterol 65 mg; Sodium 75 mg

STORAGE

Room Temperature: **airtight container, 2 days**

Refrigerator: **airtight container, 4 days**

Ancient Grain Angel Food Cake

The same moist, light and chewy texture you'd expect in any other
angel food cake, but with coconut and sorghum flours for extra nutrition.
We like to save the unused egg yolks for custards, crème brûlée or puddings.

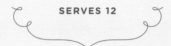

SERVES 12

Set the oven rack to its lowest position. Preheat the oven to 350°F (180°C). Set aside a 10-inch (4 L) ungreased tube pan.

Place the tapioca starch, coconut and sorghum flours and ½ cup (125 mL) of the sugar in a medium bowl and mix to combine. Set aside.

Beat the egg whites in a large bowl. When peaks are starting to form, add the cream of tartar, salt, vanilla and almond extract. Slowly add in the remaining ½ cup (125 mL) sugar and continue to beat until stiff peaks form. Slowly fold in small portions of the flour mixture and stir, using a large spoon or spatula. Scoop the mixture into the tube pan. Use a spatula or knife to cut through the batter to remove any large air pockets.

Bake for 55 minutes to 1 hour, until the cake is golden brown, the top springs back when touched and the edges have begun to pull away from the sides of the pan. Remove the cake from the oven and immediately invert it over the neck of a bottle or a funnel (even right onto a plate is fine). Leave the cake inverted, in the pan, to cool completely. Remove from the pan and cut into slices.

PER SERVING: Energy 120 calories; Protein 4 g; Carbohydrates 25 g; Dietary Fiber 1 g; Fat 0.5 g; Sugar 17 g; Cholesterol 0 mg; Sodium 110 mg

½ cup (125 mL) tapioca starch

¼ cup (60 mL) coconut flour

¼ cup (60 mL) sorghum flour

1 cup (250 mL) organic cane sugar, separated

12 large egg whites, at room temperature

2 tsp (10 mL) cream of tartar

¼ tsp (1 mL) salt

2 tsp (10 mL) pure vanilla extract

1 tsp (5 mL) pure almond extract

BAKING TIP

· Not greasing the tube pan allows the angel food cake to climb and rise in the pan.

· Inverting the cake over a bottle while cooling prevents the cake from falling too much.

STORAGE

Room Temperature: **airtight container, 2 days**
Refrigerator: **airtight container, 4 days**

Fluffy White Quinoa Cake

Chocolate cake, move over! This angelic white cake has a light fluffy crumb and is just begging to be decorated! Unobtrusive fluffy cooked quinoa seeds make this cake ultra-moist. We can guarantee that those eating it won't know they are eating ancient grains. This is even better the next day. (Save the unused egg yolks for custards or other egg-based desserts.)

SERVES 12

⅔ cup (150 mL) white or golden quinoa seeds

1 ⅓ cups (325 mL) 1% milk or light-flavored milk substitute

⅔ cup (150 mL) unsalted butter, melted and cooled, or virgin coconut oil

6 large egg whites

2 Tbsp (30 mL) pure vanilla extract

1 ¼ cups (310 mL) organic cane sugar

½ cup (125 mL) sorghum flour

¼ cup (60 mL) oat flour

¾ cup (175 mL) white rice flour

1 Tbsp (15 mL) baking powder

1 tsp (5 mL) psyllium husks

½ tsp (2 mL) salt

Preheat the oven to 375°F (190°C). Lightly grease two 9-inch (1.5 L) round cake pans. Place parchment paper in the bottom of each and lightly grease the parchment.

Place the quinoa in a small saucepan with 1 ⅓ cups (325 mL) of water and bring to a boil. Turn down the heat to a simmer, cover the saucepan and cook for 15 minutes. Remove from the heat and keep covered for an additional 15 minutes (the quinoa should be fully cooked, plump and fluffy). Let cool.

Place 2 cups (500 mL) of the cooked quinoa in a blender with the milk, butter, egg whites and vanilla. Puree until completely smooth. Set aside.

Whisk together the sugar, sorghum, oat and rice flours, baking powder, psyllium and salt in a large bowl. Add the blended quinoa mixture and stir until combined. Divide the batter between the two cake pans.

Bake for 35 to 40 minutes, until a toothpick inserted in the center comes out clean. Cool completely before frosting with Whipped Yogurt Frosting (page 84) or a double batch of marshmallow cream from the Chocolate Whoopie Pies recipe (page 21).

PER SERVING: Energy 240 calories; Protein 6 g; Carbohydrates 36 g; Dietary Fiber 2 g; Fat 10 g; Sugar 17 g; Cholesterol 25 mg; Sodium 125 mg

STORAGE

Room Temperature: airtight container or bag, 1 day

Refrigerator: airtight container or bag, 4 days

Freezer: unfrosted in an airtight freezer bag, 2 weeks

Cinnamon Apple Coffee Cake

This golden, fluffy, moist coffee cake has the perfect amount of sweetness. Oat, quinoa and sorghum flours make this cake light and airy — and definitely yummy. Honeycrisp and Granny Smith apples both work well in this recipe, but use your favorite type of baking apple.

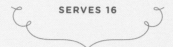

SERVES 16

Lightly grease or spray with cooking oil a 9-inch (2.5 L) square baking pan. Line the pan with parchment paper. Preheat the oven to 350°F (180°C).

Place the oat, quinoa and sorghum flours, tapioca starch, baking powder, baking soda, salt, cinnamon and nutmeg in a medium bowl and mix well to combine. Toss in the apples and walnuts and coat them evenly. Set aside.

In a separate medium bowl, mix the yogurt and oil together, then add the eggs one at a time. Add the sugars and vanilla, and mix well to combine. Add the yogurt and egg mixture to the flour mixture and mix well — but don't overmix. Pour the batter evenly into the prepared pan.

Bake for 40 to 45 minutes, until the top springs back when gently pressed or a toothpick inserted in the center comes out with only a few small crumbs. Let cool completely in the pan.

PER SERVING: Energy 240 calories; Protein 5 g; Carbohydrates 30 g; Dietary Fiber 4 g; Fat 11 g; Sugar 14 g; Cholesterol 35 mg; Sodium 135 mg

1 cup (250 mL) oat flour

1 cup (250 mL) quinoa flour

½ cup (125 mL) sorghum flour

½ cup (125 mL) tapioca starch

2 tsp (10 mL) baking powder

½ tsp (2 mL) baking soda

½ tsp (2 mL) salt

1 tsp (5 mL) cinnamon

¼ tsp (1 mL) nutmeg

3 cups (750 mL) peeled, chopped apples

½ cup (125 mL) finely chopped walnuts

1 cup (250 mL) 0% plain Greek yogurt

½ cup (125 mL) grapeseed or organic light-tasting oil

3 large eggs

½ cup (125 mL) lightly packed brown sugar

½ cup (125 mL) organic cane sugar

2 tsp (10 mL) pure vanilla extract

STORAGE
Room Temperature: airtight container, 1-2 days
Refrigerator: airtight container, 2-3 days

Coconut Cake with Whipped Yogurt Frosting

This white, luxurious cake makes a stunning addition to any table. A definite head-turner, it's made with virgin coconut oil, has a thick filling of Greek yogurt frosting and is topped with more frosting and a sprinkling of coconut.

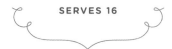

SERVES 16

CAKE

⅔ cup (150 mL) sorghum flour

½ cup (125 mL) millet flour

⅓ cup (75 mL) coconut flour

½ cup (125 mL) tapioca starch

2 tsp (10 mL) baking powder

½ tsp (2 mL) salt

1 cup (250 mL) virgin coconut oil

1 cup (250 mL) coconut milk

¾ cup (175 mL) organic
   cane sugar

4 large eggs

FROSTING

1 ½ cups (375 mL) thick, Greek
   nonfat yogurt

⅔ cup (150 mL) powdered
   (icing) sugar

½ tsp (2 mL) coconut extract

¼ cup (60 mL) unsweetened
   medium-shredded coconut

Lightly grease two 8-inch (2 L) round cake pans. Line the bottom of each pan with parchment paper. Preheat the oven to 350°F (180°C).

For the cake, place the sorghum, millet and coconut flours, tapioca starch, baking powder and salt in a medium bowl and mix to combine. Set aside.

In a separate bowl, cream the coconut oil and coconut milk with the sugar and eggs. Stir the coconut oil mixture into the flour mixture. Pour the batter evenly into the prepared pans.

Bake for 25 to 30 minutes, until the middle of the cakes spring back when gently pressed or a toothpick inserted in the center comes out with only a few small crumbs. Let the cakes cool completely in the pans.

For the frosting, beat the Greek yogurt, powdered sugar and coconut extract with an electric mixer in a medium bowl until well blended.

Place one cake on a flat plate or cake plate and spread the top with a layer of yogurt frosting. Place the other cake on top. Cover the entire cake with frosting and sprinkle with coconut. Chill for at least 1 hour before serving. This can be made the night before you plan to serve it.

PER SERVING: Energy 280 calories; Protein 5 g; Carbohydrates 27 g; Dietary Fiber 2 g; Fat 17 g; Sugar 15 g; Cholesterol 45 mg; Sodium 110 mg

STORAGE

Refrigerator: **airtight container, 3 days**

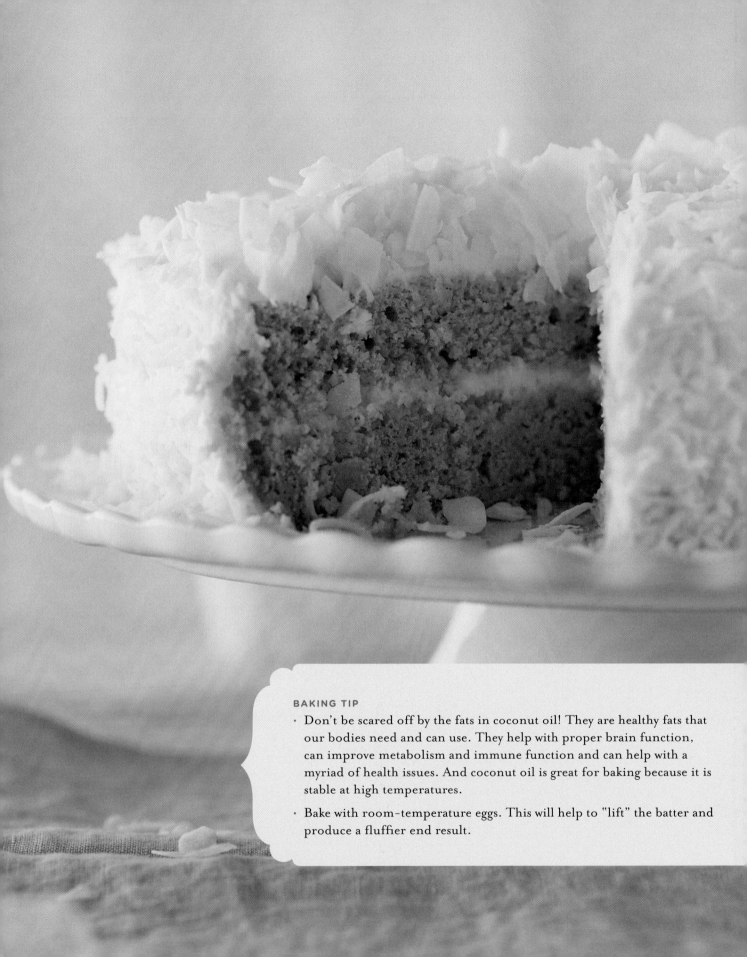

BAKING TIP

· Don't be scared off by the fats in coconut oil! They are healthy fats that our bodies need and can use. They help with proper brain function, can improve metabolism and immune function and can help with a myriad of health issues. And coconut oil is great for baking because it is stable at high temperatures.

· Bake with room-temperature eggs. This will help to "lift" the batter and produce a fluffier end result.

Lemon Crêpe Cake

Layer upon layer of tangy lemon sandwiched between tender crêpes will have you sneaking back to the refrigerator for more. Make the crêpes the day before you plan to serve this, then easily assemble the dish with layers of lemon filling and a topping of whipped cream and blackberries. Delicious on the day it is made, it is even better the day after! Use whipped coconut cream instead of whipped cream, if desired (page 124).

SERVES 16

CRÊPES

½ cup (125 mL) light buckwheat flour

½ cup (125 mL) sorghum flour

¼ cup (60 mL) white rice flour

3 Tbsp (45 mL) cornstarch

6 large eggs

2 cups (500 mL) 1% milk

⅓ cup (75 mL) liquid honey

1 ½ tsp (7 mL) pure vanilla extract

LEMON FILLING

1 cup (250 mL) liquid honey

1 cup (250 mL) fresh lemon juice (4 to 5 lemons)

¼ cup (60 mL) cornstarch

pinch salt

3 large eggs, lightly beaten

4 tsp (20 mL) lemon zest

2 Tbsp (30 mL) unsalted butter

TOPPING

1 cup (250 mL) chilled whipping cream

1-2 Tbsp (15-30 mL) organic cane sugar

½ tsp (2 mL) pure vanilla extract

1 cup (250 mL) fresh blackberries (or blueberries)

For the crêpes, place the buckwheat, sorghum and rice flours in a small bowl with the cornstarch. Mix to combine and set aside.

In a separate large bowl, whisk together the eggs, milk, honey and vanilla. Slowly add the flour mixture to the egg mixture and stir until well mixed.

Lightly spray with cooking oil or grease and preheat an 8-inch (20 cm) crêpe pan on medium-high heat. Pour 3 Tbsp (45 mL) of batter into the center of the pan (using a ¼ cup/60 mL measuring cup to help you measure); quickly tilt the pan in a circular motion to evenly spread the batter over the bottom, forming a circle the same size as the bottom of the pan. Flip the crêpe when the edges begin to curl, about 30 seconds. Cook the other side for 30 seconds, then remove from the pan. Place the hot crêpe on a plate and cover with aluminum foil. Repeat with the remaining batter, piling the crêpes one on top of the other. This batter will make 18 to 20 crêpes. Set the cooked crêpes aside.

For the filling, place the honey, lemon juice, cornstarch and salt in a medium saucepan with 1 cup (250 mL) of water. Whisk in the eggs. Bring to a full simmer over medium-low heat. Simmer for 1 minute, or until thickened enough to coat the back of a spoon. Remove from the heat. Stir in the lemon zest and butter. Allow to cool to room temperature.

Spread about 2 Tbsp (30 mL) of lemon filling evenly over each crêpe. Repeat with the remaining crêpes, leaving a bare one on top. Cover with plastic wrap and refrigerate for at least 2 hours.

For the topping, whip the cream, sugar and vanilla together until soft peaks form. Prior to serving, spread the top of the cake with the cream and top with berries. To serve, simply slice as you would any cake.

PER SERVING: Energy 260 calories; Protein 6 g; Carbohydrates 38 g; Dietary Fiber 2 g; Fat 9 g; Sugar 21 g; Cholesterol 125 mg; Sodium 60 mg

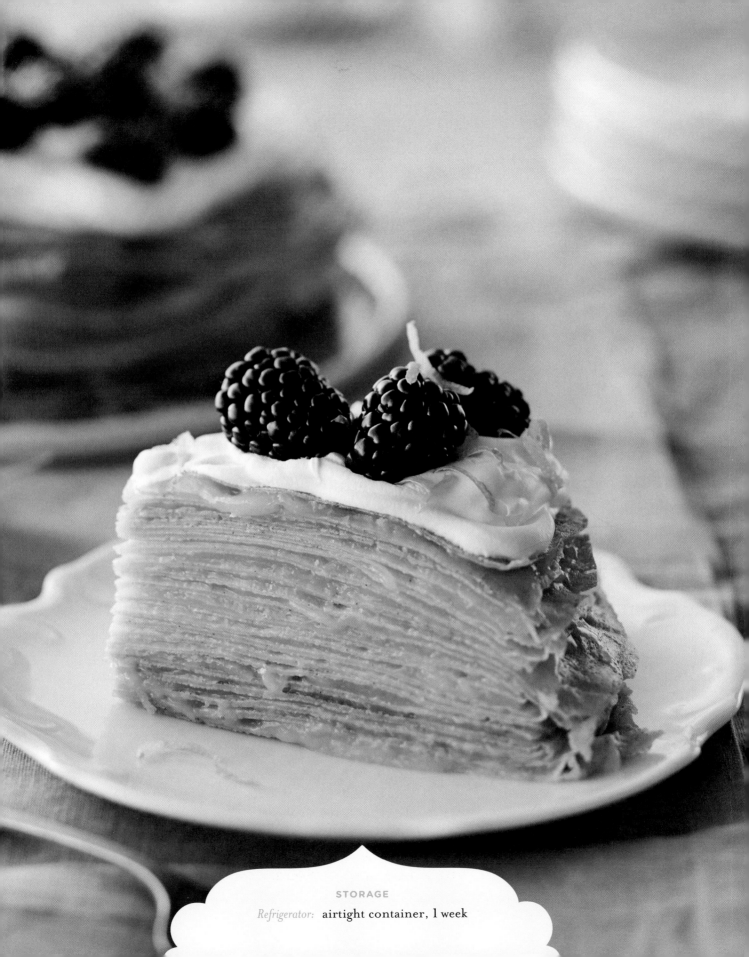

Chocolate Cream Cheese Coconut Cake

This delicious, rich-tasting cake is great for guests, especially children or anyone with a sweet tooth. It is a very moist, fluffy chocolate cake topped with cream cheese, coconut, walnuts and extra chocolate.

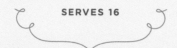

SERVES 16

½ cup (125 mL) teff flour

½ cup (125 mL) sorghum flour

¼ cup (60 mL) oat flour

½ cup (125 mL) unsweetened
sifted cocoa powder

½ cup (125 mL) organic
cane sugar

2 ½ tsp (12 mL) baking powder

½ tsp (2 mL) baking soda

½ tsp (2 mL) salt

1 large egg

1 cup (250 mL) 0% plain
Greek yogurt

¾ cup (175 mL) 1% or 2% milk
or milk substitute

1 tsp (5 mL) pure vanilla extract

⅓ cup (75 mL) virgin coconut oil

8 oz (250 g) package plain cream
cheese, softened

2 Tbsp (30 mL) unsalted butter,
softened

¾ cup (175 mL) powdered
(icing) sugar

½ cup (125 mL) unsweetened
shredded coconut

½ cup (125 mL) chopped walnuts
or pecans

½ cup (125 mL) semisweet
chocolate chips

STORAGE

Room Temperature: **airtight container or bag, 4 days**

Lightly spray with cooking oil or grease a 9-inch (2.5 L) square baking pan. Line the pan with parchment paper. Preheat the oven to 400°F (200°C).

Place the teff, sorghum and oat flours, cocoa, cane sugar, baking powder, baking soda and salt in a medium bowl and mix well to combine. Set aside.

In a separate large bowl, mix together the egg, yogurt, milk and vanilla. Mix well and add to the flour mixture, stirring until just combined. Pour into the prepared baking pan and set aside.

In another bowl, beat the coconut oil with the cream cheese, butter and powdered sugar. Place this mixture in heaping spoonfuls on top of the chocolate cake batter. Using a knife, draw a few lines through the cream cheese mixture to incorporate it slightly. Scatter coconut and walnuts evenly overtop. Lastly, top with chocolate chips.

Bake for 30 to 35 minutes, until a toothpick inserted in the center comes out with only one or two crumbs. Remove the cake from the oven and allow to cool completely in the pan.

PER SERVING: Energy 260 calories; Protein 6 g; Carbohydrates 27 g; Dietary Fiber 3 g; Fat 14 g; Sugar 16 g; Cholesterol 25 mg; Sodium 190 mg.

BAKING TIP

· To suit your tastes, or to use up whatever you have in the kitchen for gluten-free flour, use any combinations of oat, millet, sorghum, quinoa, arrowroot or light buckwheat flours.

· Always use fresh nuts! Often allergic reactions to nuts may be caused by mold. Reduce the chances of this and ensure the flavor of your recipes is not compromised by using the freshest nuts you can find and store them in sealed containers with their original packaging or labeled with their best-before dates. Always double-check the expiry date on the package before you buy! Avoid bulk-buying nuts, as freshness and expiry dates cannot be guaranteed.

Devil's Food Cake

Indulge in this devilishly dense chocolate cake made from one of our favorite gluten-free flour blends of sorghum, teff and oats. This is perfect served with a drizzle of chocolate sauce or raspberry coulis.

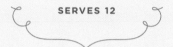

SERVES 12

³/₄ cup (175 mL) oat flour

¹/₂ cup (125 mL) teff flour

¹/₂ cup (125 mL) sorghum flour

¹/₄ cup (60 mL) tapioca starch

1 tsp (5 mL) baking powder

1 tsp (5 mL) baking soda

5 oz (140 g) unsweetened
   baking chocolate

¹/₄ cup (60 mL) grapeseed
   or virgin coconut oil

¹/₃ cup (75 mL) unsweetened
   applesauce

3 large eggs

1 cup (250 mL) lightly packed
   brown sugar

1 cup (250 mL) buttermilk
   (or milk-vinegar substitute)

2 tsp (10 mL) pure vanilla extract

2 Tbsp (30 mL) powdered
   (icing) sugar

Lightly grease or spray with cooking oil a 9-inch (2.5 L) tube pan or Bundt pan. Preheat the oven to 350°F (180°C).

Place the oat, teff and sorghum flours, tapioca starch, baking powder and baking soda in a medium bowl and mix to combine. Set aside.

Melt the chocolate over low heat in a double boiler. When almost all the chocolate is melted, remove from the heat and stir until it is completely melted. Set aside.

Mix the oil with the applesauce in a medium bowl, then beat in the eggs one at a time. Add the brown sugar, buttermilk, vanilla and ¼ cup (60 mL) of water. Stir in the melted chocolate. Add the chocolate mixture to the flour mixture, stirring until just combined. Pour the batter evenly into the prepared pan.

Bake for 50 to 55 minutes, until the top springs back when gently pressed or a toothpick inserted in the center comes out clean. Let cool completely in the pan. Lightly dust with powdered sugar, or frost with the frosting from the Outrageous Quinoa Chocolate Cake (page 91), if desired. If frosting, refrigerate for 2 hours first.

PER SERVING: Energy 250 calories; Protein 6 g; Carbohydrates 32 g; Dietary Fiber 4 g; Fat 13 g; Sugar 15 g; Cholesterol 50 mg; Sodium 150 mg

STORAGE
Room Temperature: **airtight container or bag, 1-2 days**

Outrageous Quinoa Chocolate Cake

A version of this first appeared in our book Quinoa 365: The Everyday Superfood, *but this version is even healthier and has enhanced flavor! Bake this dense, fudgy cake for your next social event. No one would guess that it's not Grandma's. Made with nutritious cooked and pureed quinoa seeds, this super-delicious chocolate cake will amaze you.*

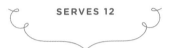

SERVES 12

Lightly grease or spray with cooking oil two 8-inch (2 L) round cake pans. Line the bottoms with parchment paper. Lightly dust the insides of the pans with cocoa. Preheat the oven to 350°F (180°C).

For the cake, bring the coffee and quinoa to a boil in a medium saucepan. Turn down the heat to a simmer, cover and cook for 15 minutes. Remove from the heat. Keep covered for an additional 15 minutes (the quinoa should be fully cooked and fluffy).

Place 2 cups (500 mL) of the cooked quinoa in a blender with the eggs, butter, milk, oil and vanilla. Puree until completely smooth.

In a medium bowl, whisk the sugar with the cocoa, psyllium, baking powder, baking soda and salt. Add the contents of the blender to the cocoa mixture and stir until thoroughly combined. Divide the batter equally between the pans.

Bake for 40 to 45 minutes, or until a toothpick inserted in the center comes out clean. Let cool completely in the pans.

While the cake cools, prepare the frosting. Ensure you open the coconut milk can from the top (that is, not the end it was standing on in the refrigerator). Pour off the coconut water into a jar to use for smoothies later (you can also freeze it in an ice cube tray). Scoop out the coconut cream from the can. It should be as thick as butter.

Continued

CAKE

1 ⅓ cups (325 mL) cold coffee

⅔ cup (150 mL) white or golden quinoa seeds

4 large eggs

½ cup (125 mL) unsalted butter, melted

⅓ cup (75 mL) 1% milk or milk substitute

¼ cup (60 mL) grapeseed or organic light-tasting oil

1 tsp (5 mL) pure vanilla extract

1 cup (250 mL) organic cane sugar

⅔ cup (150 mL) unsweetened cocoa powder, plus 2 Tbsp (30 mL) for dusting

2 tsp (10 mL) psyllium husks

1 ½ tsp (7 mL) baking powder

½ tsp (2 mL) baking soda

½ tsp (2 mL) salt

FROSTING

13.5 oz (398 mL) can full-fat coconut milk, chilled for at least 8 hours, or 1 cup (250 mL) whipping cream, chilled

1 cup (250 mL) milk chocolate chips

TOPPING

fresh blueberries

Heat 1 cup (250 mL) of the coconut cream almost to a simmer in a small saucepan. Remove from the heat and stir in the chocolate until completely melted. Pour into a bowl in preparation for whipping. Cover and chill in the refrigerator for 2 hours, until cold. Whip the chocolate mixture on medium-high until fluffy, thick and stiff peaks form. Place one cake layer on a plate and spread with one-quarter of the frosting. Top with the second cake and use the remaining frosting to cover. Scatter fresh blueberries overtop before serving.

PER SERVING: Energy 380 calories; Protein 6 g; Carbohydrates 34 g; Dietary Fiber 3 g; Fat 20 g; Sugar 24 g; Cholesterol 85 mg; Sodium 190 mg

BAKING TIP

· Replace ¼ cup (60 mL) of the butter with ¼ cup (60 mL) of mashed banana to reduce the fat content.

· When buying coconut milk for the frosting, only buy cans where the ingredients are coconut solids/cream and water. Do not use coconut milk that contains other ingredients, as additional stabilizers and preservatives can prevent the frosting from forming properly.

STORAGE

Room Temperature: airtight container, 2 days
Refrigerator: airtight container or bag, 1 week
Freezer: unfrosted in an airtight freezer bag, 2 weeks

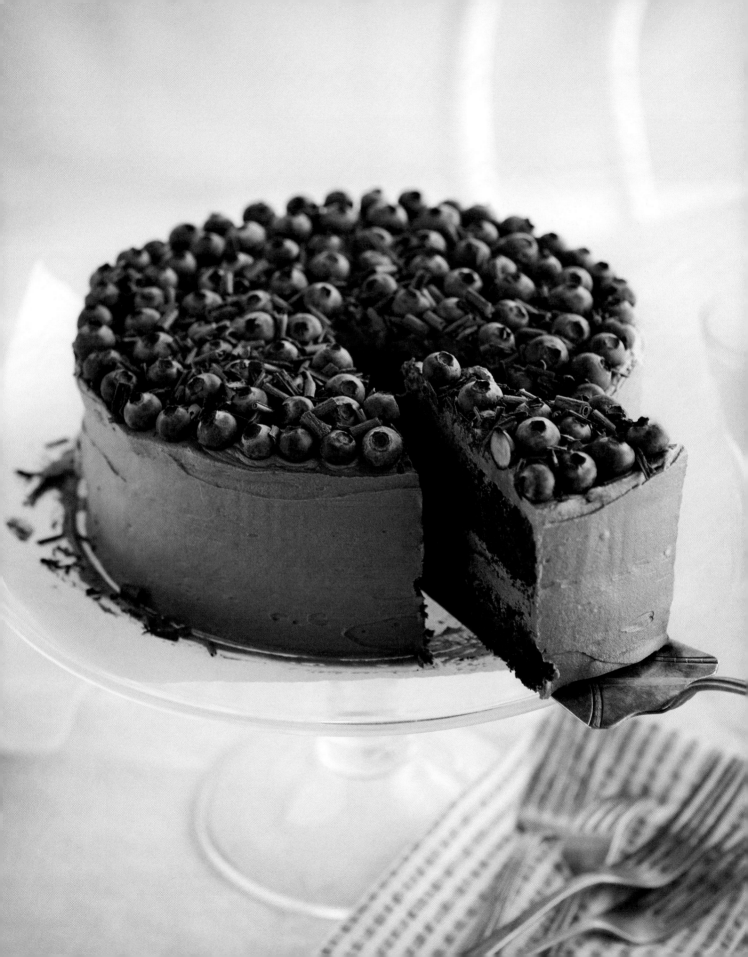

Blackberry Honey Clafoutis

We've taken this traditional, pancake-like dessert and made it with oat and sorghum flours and plenty of antioxidant-rich blackberries to make it undeniably delicious and more nutritious.

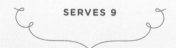

SERVES 9

2 cups (500 mL) fresh
blackberries

⅓ cup (75 mL) sorghum flour

⅓ cup (75 mL) oat flour

¼ cup (60 mL) tapioca starch

½ tsp (2 mL) cinnamon

pinch salt

3 large eggs

¼ cup (60 mL) lightly packed
brown sugar

¼ cup (60 mL) organic
cane sugar

¼ cup (60 mL) buttermilk

¼ cup (60 mL) liquid honey

2 tsp (10 mL) pure vanilla extract

Lightly spray with cooking oil or grease an 8-inch (2 L) square baking pan. Line the pan with parchment paper. Preheat the oven to 350°F (180°C).

Arrange the blackberries evenly in a single layer in the bottom of the pan and set aside.

Place the sorghum flour, oat flour, tapioca starch, cinnamon and salt in a medium bowl and mix to combine. Set aside.

In a separate large bowl, mix the eggs with the sugars, buttermilk, honey and vanilla. Add this to the flour mixture, mixing just to combine. Pour into the prepared baking pan overtop the berries.

Bake for 38 to 40 minutes, until the edges are slightly golden and a toothpick inserted in the center comes out with only one or two crumbs. Remove the cake from the oven and allow to cool slightly in the pan before serving.

PER SERVING: Energy 160 calories; Protein 4 g; Carbohydrates 31 g; Dietary Fiber 3 g; Fat 2.5 g; Sugar 17 g; Cholesterol 65 mg; Sodium 65 mg

BAKING TIP
Be sure to use fresh blackberries in this recipe. Frozen will introduce extra moisture, which will make the cake wet and mushy.

STORAGE
Refrigerator: airtight container, 3 days

Raisin Farmhouse Pudding

This was inspired by a vintage farmhouse recipe more than a century old. Back then, what you baked depended on what ingredients you had in the cupboard. This yummy cake, baked with plump raisins, caramel and vanilla, is hard to resist. Serve cold or warm, with or without ice cream.

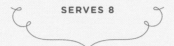

SERVES 8

Lightly spray with cooking oil or grease a 9-inch (2.5 L) square baking dish. Preheat the oven to 375°F (190°C).

For the sauce, place the sugar, raisins and butter in a medium saucepan with 2 cups (500 mL) of water and simmer until the sugar has dissolved, 3 to 5 minutes. Remove from the heat and add the vanilla. Stir, then set aside.

For the cake, mix together the sorghum flour, tapioca starch, sugar, baking powder and xanthan gum in a medium bowl. Work in the cold butter with a pastry cutter until the butter is in small pieces. Pour in the milk and vanilla and work together, using a spoon or your hands, until a dough is formed. Flatten the dough evenly across the bottom of the baking dish, keeping it ¼ inch (0.5 cm) from the edges. Pour the hot raisin mixture over the dough.

Bake for 25 to 30 minutes, or until a toothpick inserted in the center of the cake comes out clean. Let rest for 10 minutes before serving.

PER SERVING: Energy 240 calories; Protein 2 g; Carbohydrates 45 g; Dietary Fiber 4 g; Fat 5 g; Sugar 21 g; Cholesterol 10 mg; Sodium 20 mg

SAUCE

⅔ cup (150 mL) lightly packed brown sugar

½ cup (125 mL) seedless raisins

1 Tbsp (15 mL) unsalted butter

1 tsp (5 mL) pure vanilla extract

CAKE

¾ cup (175 mL) sorghum flour

¾ cup (175 mL) tapioca starch

3 Tbsp (45 mL) organic cane sugar

2 tsp (10 mL) baking powder

½ tsp (2 mL) xanthan gum

2 Tbsp (30 mL) cold unsalted butter

½ cup (125 mL) 1% or 2% milk or milk substitute

1 tsp (5 mL) pure vanilla extract

STORAGE

Refrigerator: **airtight container, 2 days**

Pineapple Citrus Berry Crisp

Juicy pineapple with star anise, brown sugar and a dash of berries and citrus make this sorghum, oat and millet ancient grain crisp burst with diverse, complementary flavors.

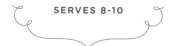

SERVES 8-10

FILLING

1 whole pineapple, trimmed and chopped

1 cup (250 mL) raspberries, frozen or fresh

2 Tbsp (30 mL) lightly packed brown sugar

1 Tbsp (15 mL) fresh lemon juice

1 Tbsp (15 mL) lemon zest

½ tsp (2 mL) anise seed

TOPPING

¾ cup (175 mL) old-fashioned rolled oats

½ cup (125 mL) sorghum flour

¼ cup (60 mL) millet flour

⅓ cup (75 mL) lightly packed brown sugar

¼ tsp (1 mL) cinnamon

⅓ cup (75 mL) melted unsalted butter

Lightly spray with cooking oil or grease a 9-inch (2 L) square baking pan or an 11- × 7-inch (2 L) baking pan or dish. Preheat the oven to 375°F (190°C).

For the filling, place the pineapple chunks and raspberries in a large bowl. Add the brown sugar, lemon juice and zest and anise seed and toss until all the ingredients are evenly distributed. Place the fruit in the prepared baking dish and set aside.

For the topping, place the oats, sorghum and millet flours, brown sugar and cinnamon in a medium bowl with the melted butter. Stir until well combined. Place the oat mixture evenly overtop the fruit mixture.

Bake for 30 to 35 minutes, until the edges of the topping turn golden brown and the filling is bubbling.

PER SERVING: Energy 190 calories; Protein 3 g; Carbohydrates 31 g; Dietary Fiber 4 g; Fat 7 g; Sugar 16 g; Cholesterol 15 mg; Sodium 5 mg

STORAGE

Refrigerator: **airtight container, 2 days**

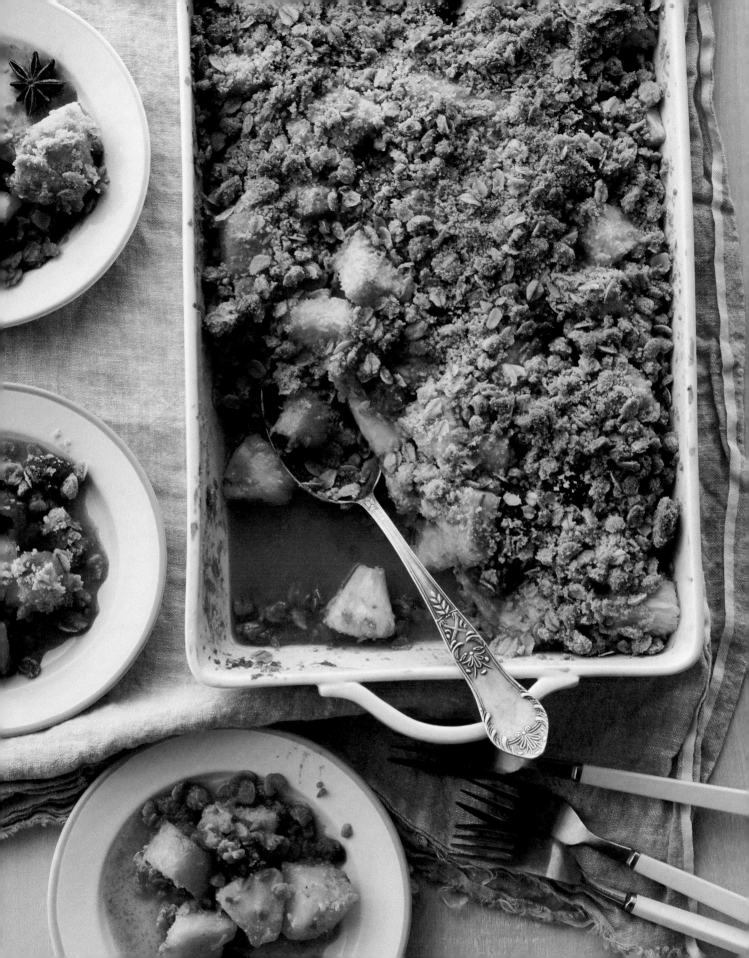

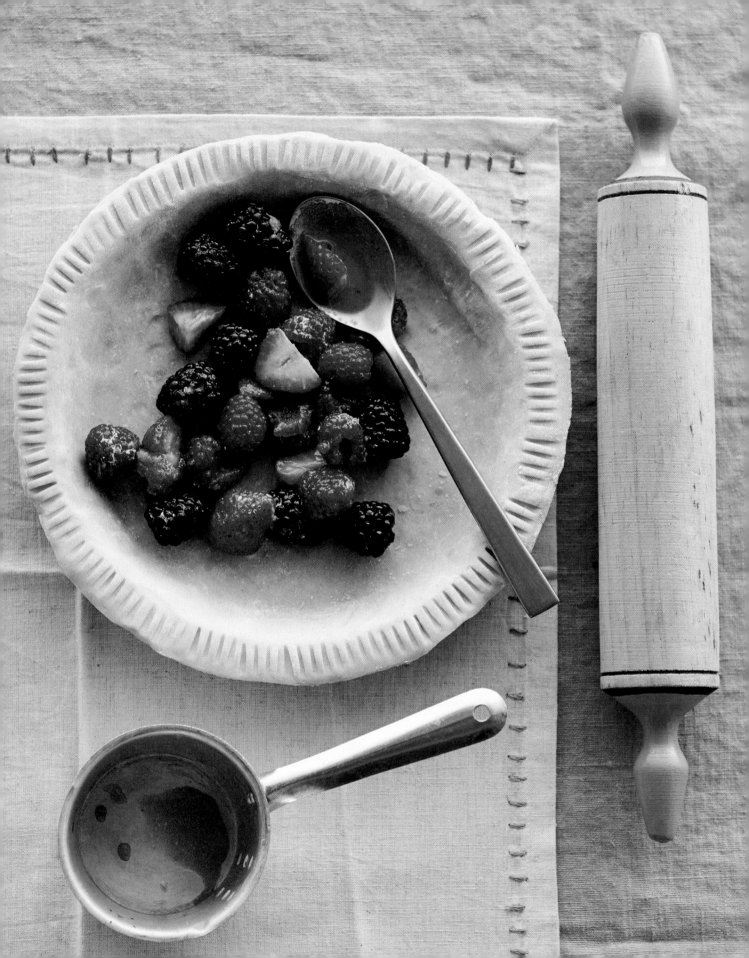

Tarts and Pies

Gluten-Free Pie Pastry I   102

Gluten-Free Pie Pastry II   103

Cream Cheese Pastry   104

Pressed Nut Crust   105

Graham-Style Wafer Crumb Crust   108

Lemon Quinoa Cream Pie   109

Caramel Apple Tarte Tatin   111

Mashed Blueberry Lime Hand Pies   112

Wild Berry Pie   114

Blueberry Goat Cheese Tart   116

Carrot Spice Pie   118

Pecan Date Pie   120

Chocolate Quinoa Pie   122

Tangy Lime Greek Yogurt Pie   124

Rich Chocolate Raspberry Tartlets   126

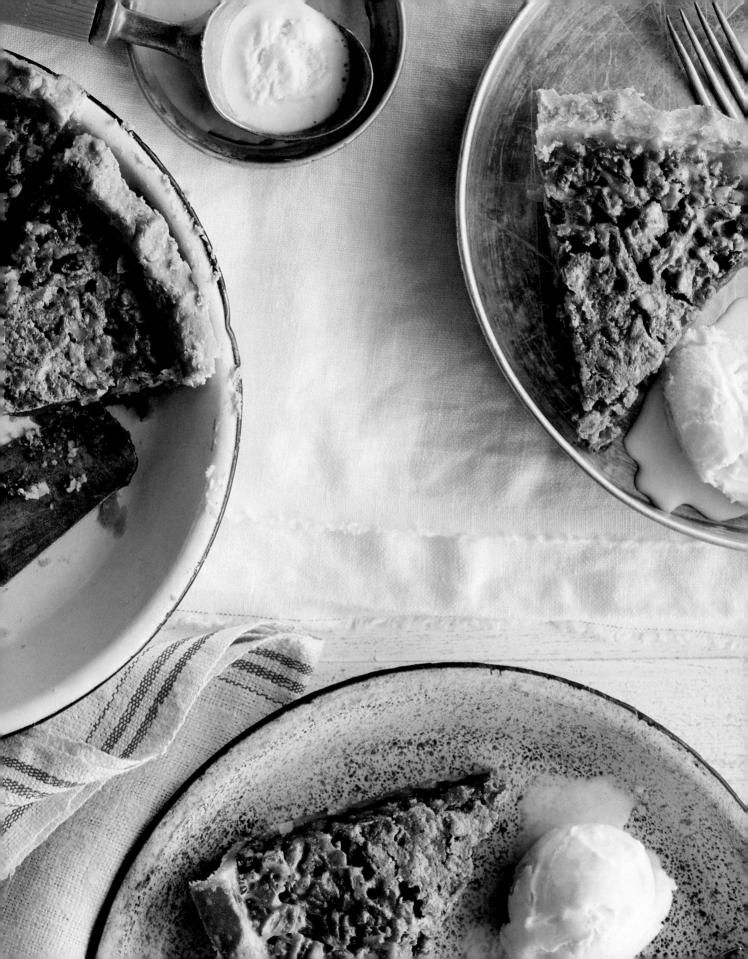

Tarts and pies are nostalgic and comforting. What could be more symbolic of a family gathering than a lovely golden baked pie? Tarts and pies are wonderful things to share with those you love after a delicious meal. Whether it's a savory meal packed in a pastry, a traditional fruit pie or a thick and creamy custard pie, pies are a reliable source of home-baked goodness. And gluten-free is just as easy with pies as with other baked goodies.

Try Gluten-Free Pie Pastry I or II (pages 102 and 103) or Cream Cheese Pastry (page 104) for basic pastry recipes, or the Pressed Nut Crust (page 105) for something completely different. Looking for a new twist on an old favorite? Try Pecan Date Pie (page 120) or the trendy individual Mashed Blueberry Lime Hand Pies (page 112) for a "handy" dessert. For a dainty dish to set before a king, feast on the Wild Berry Pie (page 114) or Tangy Lime Greek Yogurt Pie (page 124).

Gluten-Free Pie Pastry I

This simple gluten-free pastry is easy to work with and makes a light, slightly coconut-scented crust with millet and sweet sorghum flour. It's great for a variety of pies and tarts. This recipe uses coconut oil instead of butter, which we use in Gluten-Free Pie Pastry II (page 103).

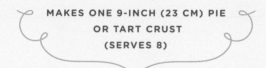

**MAKES ONE 9-INCH (23 CM) PIE
OR TART CRUST
(SERVES 8)**

½ cup (125 mL) sorghum flour

¼ cup (60 mL) millet flour

¾ cup (175 mL) tapioca starch

¼ cup (60 mL) potato
or arrowroot starch

1 tsp (5 mL) organic cane sugar

¼ tsp (1 mL) salt

½ cup (125 mL) virgin coconut oil

1 large egg

1 tsp (5 mL) apple cider vinegar

3 Tbsp (45 mL) ice water

Place the sorghum and millet flours, tapioca and potato starches, sugar and salt in a bowl and mix to combine. Using a pastry blender or two knives, cut in the coconut oil until the mixture resembles large crumbs.

In a separate bowl, whisk together the egg, vinegar and ice water. Slowly stir the egg mixture into the flour, mixing with your hands until a ball forms. Gently knead for a few minutes.

Shape the dough into a large disk and wrap it in a piece of plastic wrap. Place it in the refrigerator for 1 hour.

Have a 9-inch (23 cm) glass pie plate ready. Preheat the oven to 425°F (220°C).

Remove the dough from the refrigerator. Work it gently with your hands to soften it slightly, but keep it cold, and roll to ³⁄₁₆ inch (0.4 cm) thickness on a large piece of wax or parchment paper. Holding the dough in place, flip the paper upside down to place the dough in the center of the pie plate. To prevent bubbles or shrinking (if baking unfilled), you can prick a few holes in the pastry or cover it with a piece of parchment and put pastry weights or dried beans on top.

Bake the pastry shell for 10 to 12 minutes, until the edges are starting to turn a slight golden brown.

PER SERVING: Energy 230 calories; Protein 2 g; Carbohydrates 24 g; Dietary Fiber 1 g; Fat 11 g; Sugar 1 g; Cholesterol 25 mg; Sodium 80 mg

STORAGE
Room Temperature: airtight container, 2-3 days
Refrigerator: airtight container, 2-3 days

Gluten-Free Pie Pastry II

This traditional pastry is made gluten-free but contains butter instead of coconut oil (see Gluten-Free Pie Pastry I, page 102) for an even more neutral flavor that works well with both sweet and savory fillings.

**MAKES ONE 9-INCH (23 CM)
OR 10-INCH (25 CM) PIE OR TART CRUST
(SERVES 8)**

Place the flours, arrowroot starch, sugar and salt in a large bowl. Using a pastry blender or two knives, cut in the butter until the mixture resembles large crumbs. Using a fork, slowly stir the buttermilk into the flour mix, until a ball forms. Gently knead the dough for a few minutes.

Shape the dough into a large disk and wrap in plastic wrap. Place in the refrigerator for 1 hour.

Have a 9-inch (23 cm) or 10-inch (25 cm) glass pie plate ready. Preheat the oven to 425°F (220°C).

Remove the dough from the refrigerator and roll it to ³⁄₁₆ inch (0.4 cm) thickness on a large piece of wax or parchment paper. Holding the dough in place, flip the paper upside down to place the dough in the center of the pie plate. To prevent bubbles or shrinking (if baking unfilled), you can prick a few holes in the pastry or cover it with a piece of parchment and put pastry weights or dried beans on top.

Bake the pastry shell for 10 to 12 minutes, until the edges are starting to turn a slight golden brown.

PER SERVING: Energy 140 calories; Protein 2 g; Carbohydrates 14 g; Dietary Fiber 2 g; Fat 8 g; Sugar 2 g; Cholesterol 20 mg; Sodium 65 mg

⅓ cup (75 mL) coconut flour

⅓ cup (75 mL) sorghum flour

⅓ cup (75 mL) brown rice flour

½ cup (125 mL) arrowroot starch

1 Tbsp (15 mL) organic cane sugar

¼ tsp (1 mL) salt

½ cup (125 mL) cold unsalted butter, cubed

⅓ cup (75 mL) cold buttermilk (or cold milk-vinegar substitute)

STORAGE

Room Temperature: airtight container, 2–3 days

Refrigerator: airtight container, 2–3 days

Cream Cheese Pastry

This sturdy golden-brown crust has a flaky texture. With the slightly savory taste of cream cheese, it has a neutral enough flavor to make it suitable for everything from quiches to cream pies.

**MAKES ONE 9-INCH (23 CM)
OR 10-INCH (25 CM) PIE OR TART CRUST
(SERVES 8)**

⅓ cup (75 mL) sorghum flour

⅓ cup (75 mL) arrowroot flour
or tapioca starch

⅓ cup (75 mL) quinoa flour

1 Tbsp (15 mL) organic cane sugar

¼ tsp (1 mL) salt

4 oz (115 g) cold cream cheese
(½ package)

6 Tbsp (90 mL) cold unsalted
butter, cubed

Place the sorghum, arrowroot and quinoa flours, sugar and salt in a large bowl and mix to combine. Using a pastry blender or two knives, cut in the cream cheese and butter until the mixture resembles large crumbs. Using your hands (make sure they're cold) or a large wooden spoon, continue to mix until a ball forms. Gently knead for a few minutes.

Shape the dough into a large disk and wrap in plastic wrap. Place in the refrigerator for 1 hour.

Have a 9-inch (23 cm) or 10-inch (25 cm) glass pie plate ready. Preheat the oven to 325°F (160°C).

Remove the dough from the refrigerator and roll out to roughly ³⁄₁₆ inch (0.4 cm) thickness on a large piece of wax or parchment paper. Holding the dough in place, flip the paper upside down to place the dough in the center of the pie plate. To prevent bubbles or shrinking (if baking unfilled), you can prick a few holes in the pastry or cover it with a piece of parchment and put pastry weights or dried beans on top.

Bake the pastry shell for 25 minutes, until the edges are starting to turn a slight golden brown.

PER SERVING: Energy 190 calories; Protein 2 g; Carbohydrates 14 g; Dietary Fiber 1 g; Fat 14 g; Sugar 2 g; Cholesterol 40 mg; Sodium 120 mg

STORAGE

Room Temperature: airtight container, 1-2 days

Refrigerator: airtight container, 2-3 days

Pressed Nut Crust

*This bottom-only, pressed crust made from wholesome ground walnuts
(or pecans, if you prefer) adds another flavor dimension to your pie or tart filling.
This is excellent with any cream, pudding or fruit filling.*

MAKES ONE 9-INCH (23 CM) PIE OR TART CRUST (SERVES 8)

Place the walnuts, oat flour and chia in a medium bowl and mix to combine. Add the butter and work in until the mixture sticks together (you can use your hands for this). Add the maple syrup and continue to mix until well combined. Using your hands, press the mixture into a 9-inch (23 cm) glass pie plate. Place in the refrigerator for 1 hour.

Preheat the oven to 350°F (180°C).

Bake the crust for 13 to 15 minutes, until the outermost edges begin to turn golden brown.

PER SERVING: Energy 190 calories; Protein 4 g; Carbohydrates 11 g; Dietary Fiber 3 g; Fat 14 g; Sugar 2 g; Cholesterol 10 mg; Sodium 0 mg

1 cup (250 mL) lightly packed ground walnuts (roughly the same as the chopped amount)

1 cup (250 mL) oat flour

2 Tbsp (30 mL) ground chia seeds

3 Tbsp (45 mL) unsalted butter, softened

1 Tbsp (15 mL) pure maple syrup or liquid honey

STORAGE

Room Temperature: **airtight container, 2–3 days**

Refrigerator: **airtight container, 2–3 days**

BAKING TIP

- Similar to a crumb crust, pressed nut crusts are more crumbly than dough crusts. Before lifting a slice out of the pan, carefully run a knife around the edges to separate the crust from the dish and then cut and remove a slice. Also, cutting smaller slices will ensure they come out nice!

- Always use fresh nuts! Often allergic reactions to nuts may be caused by mold. Reduce the chance of this and ensure the flavor of your recipes is not compromised by using the freshest nuts you can find and store them in sealed containers with their original packaging or labeled with their best-before dates. Always double-check the expiry date on the package before you buy! Avoid bulk-buying nuts, as freshness and expiry dates cannot be guaranteed.

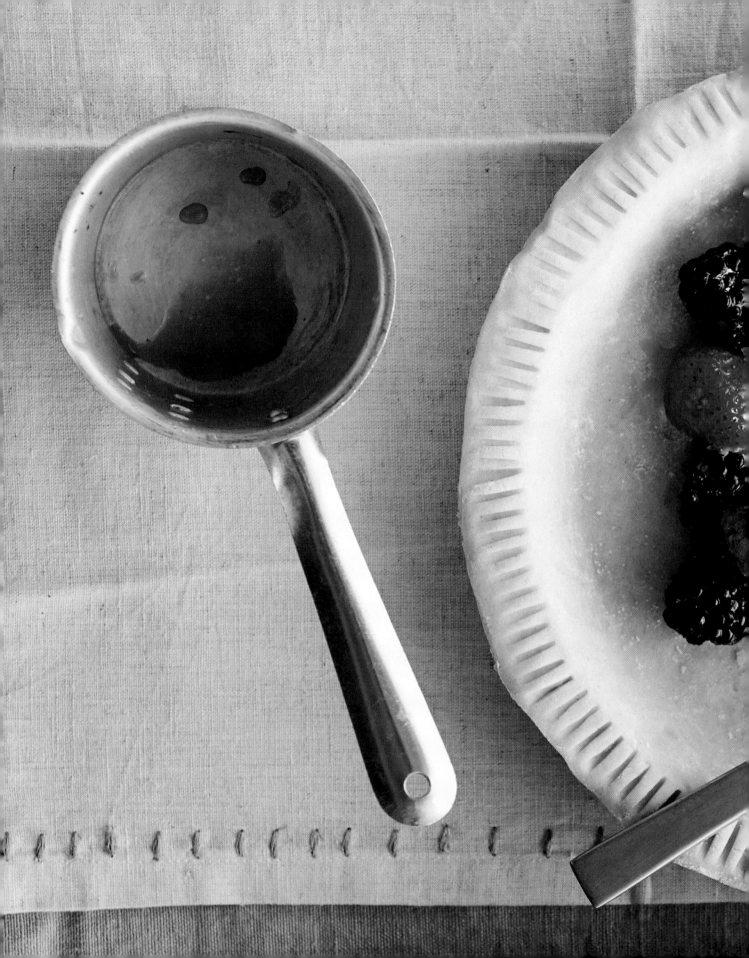

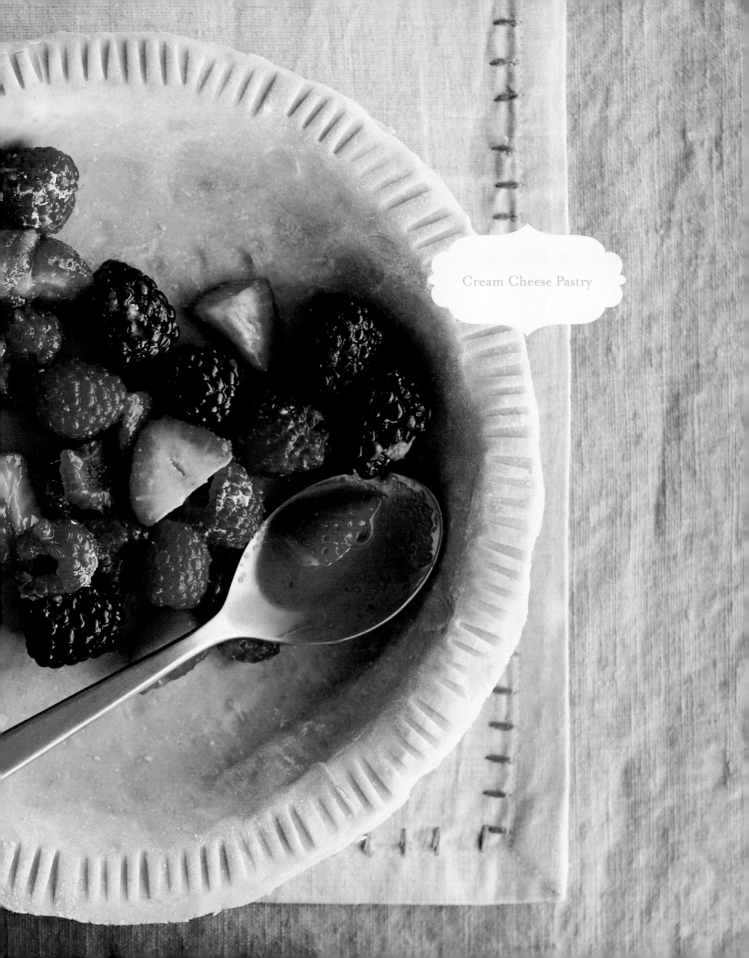

Cream Cheese Pastry

Graham-Style Wafer Crumb Crust

This graham-like wafer crumb crust makes a delicious gluten-free alternative for pudding pies, custards and cheesecakes. It needs no added sugar because the wafers already taste delicious!

**MAKES ONE 10-INCH (25 CM) PIE CRUST,
12 MUFFIN-SIZED CHEESECAKE BOTTOMS
OR 36 MINI-SIZED CHEESECAKE BOTTOMS**

1 ⅓ cups + 1 Tbsp (340 mL) crushed Graham-Style Wafers (page 46)

¼ cup (60 mL) unsalted butter, melted and cooled

Preheat the oven to 325°F (160°C).

Combine the wafer crumbs and butter in a medium bowl. Stir with a spatula until the mixture sticks together. Using your hands, press the crumbs into a 10-inch (25 cm) glass pie plate or 10-inch (3 L) springform pan (for cheesecake). If the mixture sticks to your fingers, lightly dampen your fingertips with water. Bake for 22 to 25 minutes, until lightly browned and firm. Allow to cool completely before adding any prepared pie filling.

PER SERVING (⅛ of a 10-inch/25 cm pie): Energy 110 calories; Protein 1 g; Carbohydrates 12 g; Dietary Fiber 1 g; Fat 7 g; Sugar 3 g; Cholesterol 20 mg; Sodium 45 mg

STORAGE

Refrigerator: **airtight container or bag, 3-4 days**

MUFFIN-SIZED CRUSTS

For a muffin-sized version, place 1 Tbsp (15 mL) of crumb mixture in each cup. For a mini-version, use 1 tsp (5 mL) of crumb pressed into the bottom of each cup. Paper liners are not necessary for muffin sizes, but are recommended for minis. For either size, they assist with easy removal and allow you to bake smaller batches at a time (you may not have four or five 12-cup mini-muffin pans!). Use approximately the same baking time for mini and muffin size, 8 to 10 minutes, but keep a careful watch as they bake.

BAKING TIP

The homemade wafers may cause the crust to rise a little, giving you a slightly thicker crust than you might expect. If you prefer a thinner crumb crust for a single, large cheesecake, you may want to use three-quarters of the portion of the crumb crust. (We don't recommend reducing the crust on the smaller cheesecakes.)

Lemon Quinoa Cream Pie

The tangy honey–sweet lemon pie filling is made with pureed cooked quinoa for its thickening ability and added nutrition. We recommend the Cream Cheese Pastry (page 104) for this, but feel free to use your personal favorite crust.

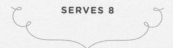

SERVES 8

Prepare the Cream Cheese Pastry crust, bake and set aside.

Place the quinoa in a medium saucepan with 2 cups (500 mL) of water. Bring to a boil, turn down the heat to a simmer, cover and cook for 25 minutes. The quinoa should be extra fluffy. Don't let it cool too much.

In a food processor or large blender, puree the cooked quinoa with the lemon juice and zest, sugar, honey, milk (if using) and salt. Puree repeatedly until the mixture is extremely smooth. If the mixture is too thick to puree, use a spatula to move it around in the blender and puree again. Pour the mixture into the cooled pastry shell. Chill in the refrigerator for 1 to 2 hours.

This is best served cold, topped with whipped cream or crème fraîche (if using).

PER SERVING: Energy 280 calories; Protein 4 g; Carbohydrates 39 g; Dietary Fiber 4 g; Fat 12 g; Sugar 18 g; Cholesterol 30 mg; Sodium 196 mg

1 recipe Cream Cheese Pastry (page 104)

1 cup (250 mL) white or golden quinoa seeds

¾ cup (175 mL) fresh lemon juice (roughly 3 lemons)

⅓ cup (75 mL) packed freshly grated lemon zest (roughly 2–3 lemons)

½ cup (125 mL) organic cane sugar

¼ cup (60 mL) liquid honey

¼ cup (60 mL) 1% or 2% milk or milk substitute (optional)

½ tsp (2 mL) salt

whipped cream or crème fraîche (optional)

BAKING TIP

· Be sure not to cool the quinoa in the refrigerator. Pureeing quinoa when it is still warm or at room temperature ensures the pie filling gels together properly into a nice thick pie.

· Avoid a bitter lemon taste by ensuring you zest only the outermost yellow of the lemon rind and do not include the bitter white pith.

· Milk makes this recipe a bit creamier, but is not essential.

STORAGE

Refrigerator: airtight container, 1–2 days

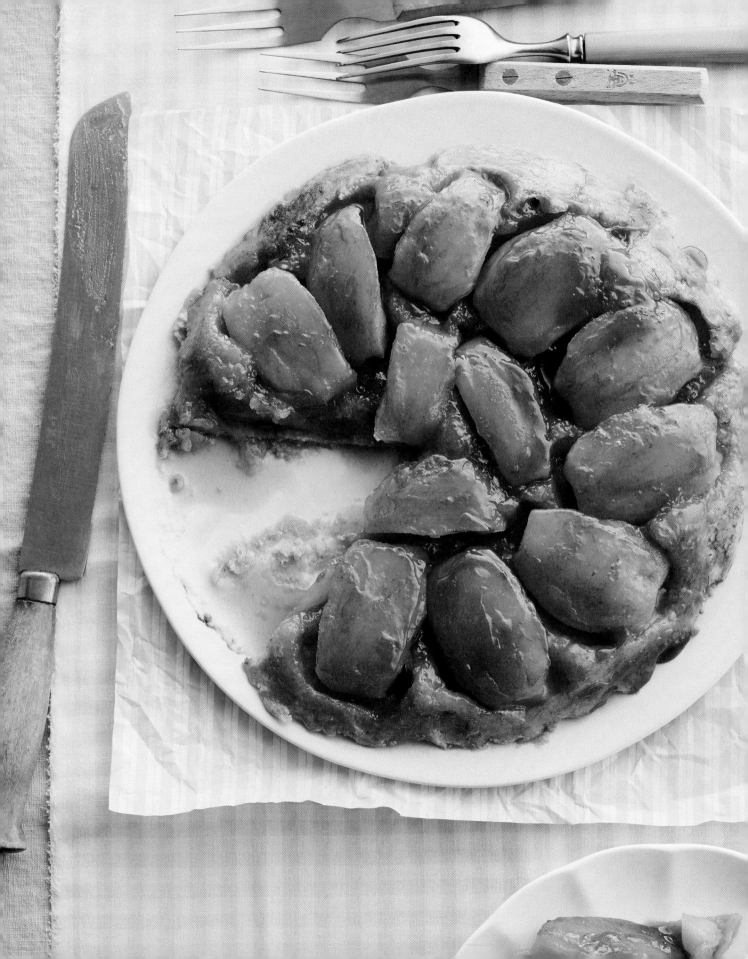

Caramel Apple Tarte Tatin

The Tatin sisters made the Tarte Tatin famous in France in the early 1900s. A traditional Tatin is a caramelized apple tart that has the pastry baked on top and is flipped for serving. Here is a healthier version (but it is also nice à la mode!).

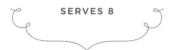

SERVES 8

Cut a piece of parchment paper approximately 12 × 12 inches (30 × 30 cm) and dust it with flour.

For the dough, place the sorghum and oat flours, tapioca starch, psyllium, sugar and salt in a bowl and whisk to combine. Cut the butter into pea-sized pieces with a pastry cutter or pinch it with your fingers. Gently stir in the cold water, a little at a time, until the dough comes together and can be easily formed into a disk. Roll the pastry out on the parchment to a circle of about 11 inches (28 cm) in diameter. Place a 10-inch (25 cm) ovenproof skillet on the dough and cut around it. Transfer the parchment and dough to a plate, cover with plastic wrap and refrigerate until cold, about 20 minutes.

Preheat the oven to 400°F (200°C).

For the apples, place the sugar and juice in the skillet you used to measure the dough circle over low heat. Simmer for 1 minute, stirring frequently. Be careful not to splash the hot sugar. Stir in the butter and simmer for another 2 minutes. Place the apple quarters snugly in the skillet in a concentric circle, slightly overlapping each other, and simmer on low heat for 9 to 10 minutes. Invert the parchment paper to place the pastry over the apples. Make three small incisions for the steam to escape.

Bake in the oven for about 20 minutes, or until the crust edges are slightly golden and juice is bubbling out from the edges. Remove from the oven and cool in the skillet for 20 minutes before turning out onto a plate and sprinkling with pecans (if using). Serve with ice cream, if desired.

PER SERVING: Energy 230 calories; Protein 1 g; Carbohydrates 32 g; Dietary Fiber 3 g; Fat 11 g; Sugar 15 g; Cholesterol 30 mg; Sodium 80 mg

DOUGH

⅓ cup (75 mL) sorghum flour

⅓ cup (75 mL) oat flour

½ cup (125 mL) tapioca starch, with extra for dusting

1 Tbsp (15 mL) psyllium husks

2 Tbsp (30 mL) organic cane sugar

¼ tsp (1 mL) salt

¼ cup (60 mL) cold unsalted butter

5–6 Tbsp (75–90 mL) cold water

APPLES

½ cup (125 mL) Sucanat or lightly packed brown sugar

¼ cup (60 mL) unsweetened apple juice

¼ cup (60 mL) unsalted butter

5 small apples (Cripps Pink or Gala), peeled, cored and quartered

2 Tbsp (30 mL) coarsely chopped, toasted pecans (optional)

STORAGE

Room Temperature: airtight container, 1 day

Refrigerator: airtight container, 5 days

Mashed Blueberry Lime Hand Pies

Handheld pies are such a treat! These beautifully rustic hand pies are tender and sweet, made with gluten-free Cream Cheese Pastry (page 104) and stuffed full of flavorful mashed blueberries scented with lime and maple syrup. Don't fret if the pies crack a bit here and there; it adds to their beauty!

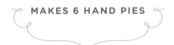

MAKES 6 HAND PIES

1 recipe Cream Cheese Pastry (page 104)

1 ½ cups (375 mL) fresh or frozen and thawed/drained blueberries

2 Tbsp (30 mL) organic cane sugar

1 Tbsp (15 mL) pure maple syrup

1 tsp (5 mL) tapioca starch

1 tsp (5 mL) fresh lime juice

½ tsp (2 mL) grated lime zest

1 large egg

1 tsp (5 mL) milk or water

Prepare the Cream Cheese Pastry, but do not roll it out or bake it. Have it ready at room temperature.

Lightly spray with cooking oil or grease a large baking sheet. Line the baking sheet with parchment paper. Preheat the oven to 375°F (190°C).

Place the blueberries, sugar, syrup, tapioca starch and lime juice and zest in a medium bowl and mix to combine. Using a potato masher or large fork, mash the mixture until no whole blueberries remain. Set aside.

On a lightly floured surface, roll out the pastry. Using a 4 ½-inch (11 cm) round cutter or tart pan, cut out six rounds of pastry. Place each one on the baking sheet. Spoon approximately 1 ½ Tbsp (22 mL) of mashed blueberry mixture into the center of each. Fold over each piece of pastry to make a half-moon shape, moisten the edges slightly with water and gently press them together. (Do not worry about small cracks in the top of the pastry, but if there's no cracking, ensure you poke a few small holes into each tart.) Mix the egg and milk together in a small bowl to make an egg wash. Brush the surface of each hand pie with this.

Bake for 20 to 22 minutes, until golden. Remove from the oven and let sit briefly to cool. Serve warm or cold.

PER SERVING: Energy 310 calories; Protein 4 g; Carbohydrates 32 g; Dietary Fiber 3 g; Fat 19 g; Sugar 1 g; Cholesterol 80 mg; Sodium 170 mg

STORAGE
Room Temperature: airtight container, 1-2 days
Refrigerator: airtight container, 3-4 days

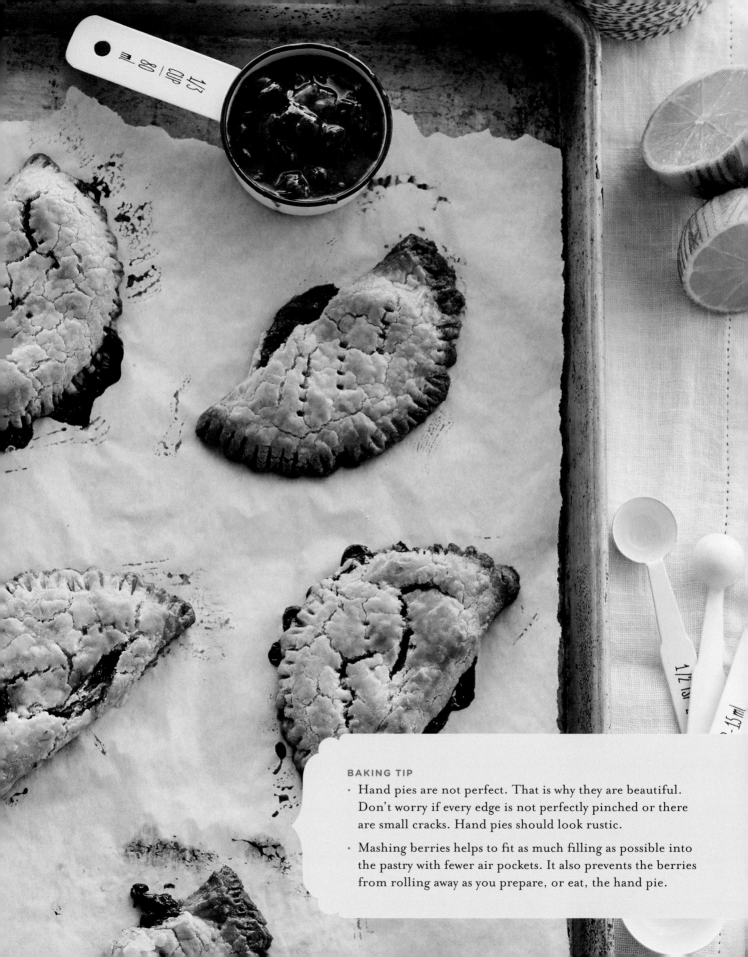

BAKING TIP

· Hand pies are not perfect. That is why they are beautiful. Don't worry if every edge is not perfectly pinched or there are small cracks. Hand pies should look rustic.

· Mashing berries helps to fit as much filling as possible into the pastry with fewer air pockets. It also prevents the berries from rolling away as you prepare, or eat, the hand pie.

Wild Berry Pie

This fresh, sweet mixed berry pie fit for a king is made with our easy Cream Cheese Pastry (page 104), which contains ancient grains. Fresh berries are required for this recipe — using frozen will introduce excess moisture, which could ruin the pie.

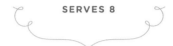

SERVES 8

double recipe Cream Cheese Pastry (page 104)

1 ½ cups (375 mL) fresh whole strawberries

1 ½ cups (375 mL) fresh blackberries

1 ½ cups (375 mL) fresh raspberries

¼ cup (60 mL) organic cane sugar

3 Tbsp (45 mL) cornstarch

1 Tbsp (15 mL) fresh lemon juice

1 Tbsp (15 mL) lemon zest

Prepare a double recipe of Cream Cheese Pastry and leave it to chill in the refrigerator until you're ready to roll it out.

Place a large baking sheet or drip tray on the bottom oven rack. Preheat the oven to 350°F (180°C).

Toss the berries in a large bowl with the sugar, cornstarch, lemon juice and zest. Set aside.

Roll out half of the pastry dough (see page 104) and place it in a 9-inch (23 cm) or 10-inch (25 cm) pie or tart plate. Place the berry mixture evenly along the bottom crust and roll out the second half of the pastry to the same size as the pie plate. Cut this piece into lattice strips, cookie cutter shapes or one large piece with holes poked in it to release the steam. Place on top of the berries.

Cover with aluminum foil and bake for 30 minutes, then remove the foil and bake for an additional 25 minutes, until the edges and top are lightly golden. Cool in the pie plate. Serve warm or cold, à la mode or plain.

PER SERVING: Energy 240 calories; Protein 3 g; Carbohydrates 29 g; Dietary Fiber 5 g; Fat 14 g; Sugar 12 g; Cholesterol 40 mg; Sodium 120 mg

STORAGE
Refrigerator: **airtight container, 2 days**

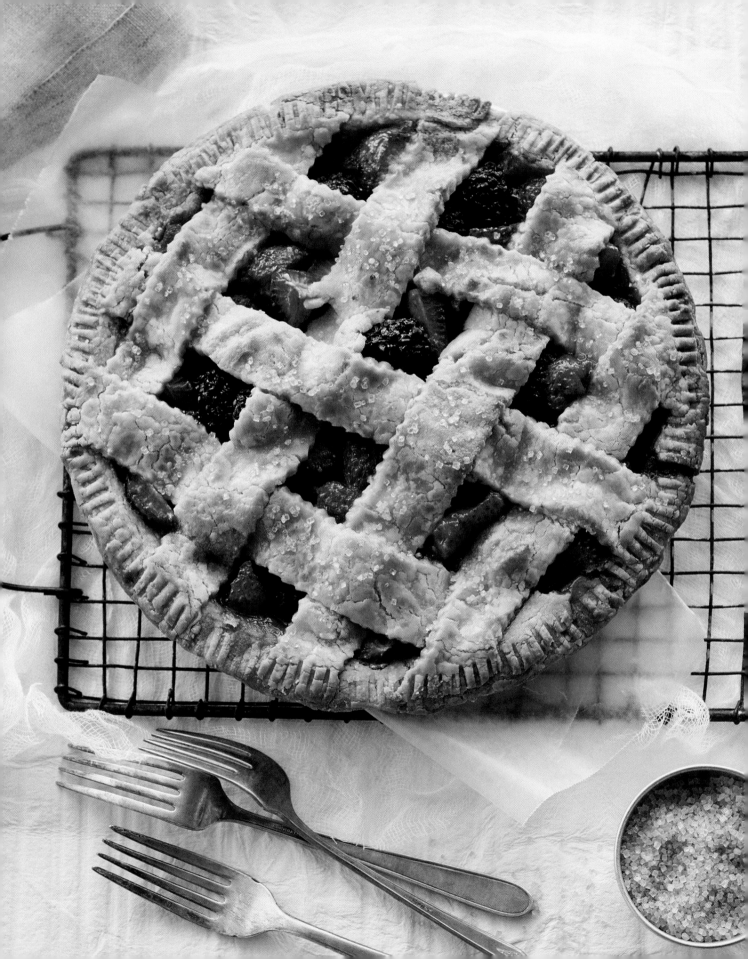

Blueberry Goat Cheese Tart

Creamy goat cheese and blueberries are a heavenly match.
Teff makes a beautiful, nutty crust that is a perfect base for this flavorful tart.

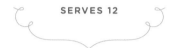 **SERVES 12**

CRUST

¾ cup (175 mL) almond flour

½ cup (125 mL) teff flour

½ tsp (2 mL) psyllium husks

⅓ cup (75 mL) lightly packed brown sugar

3 Tbsp (45 mL) unsalted butter, melted

1 large egg white, lightly beaten

FILLING

4 oz (125 g) soft, unripened goat cheese

¾ cup (75 mL) 2% plain Greek yogurt

3 Tbsp (45 mL) liquid honey

½ tsp (2 mL) pure vanilla extract

SAUCE

3 Tbsp (45 mL) liquid honey

2 ½ tsp (12 mL) cornstarch

1 ¾ cups (425 mL) frozen wild blueberries, thawed

Lightly grease a 9- or 10-inch (23-25 cm) tart pan. Preheat the oven to 350°F (180°C).

For the crust, whisk together the almond and teff flours and psyllium. Using a wooden spoon, stir in the sugar and then work in the butter, using clean hands for this stage if necessary. Stir in the egg white until fully combined. Press into the prepared tart pan. Bake for 12 minutes. Remove from the oven and let cool completely.

For the filling, place the goat cheese, yogurt, honey and vanilla in a medium mixing bowl. Use a handheld or stand mixer to mix everything fully. Spread the filling evenly over the cooled crust. Cool in the refrigerator for 45 minutes.

For the sauce, whisk the honey and cornstarch in a medium saucepan with ⅓ cup (75 mL) of water. Add the thawed blueberries. Warm the berry mixture over medium-low heat, stirring frequently until the sauce has come to a boil. Let it boil for 1 minute, until thickened enough to coat the back of a spoon. Allow the sauce to cool to room temperature, then spread it evenly over the goat cheese filling, distributing the berries evenly across the top.

Cool in the refrigerator for at least 1 hour before removing from the pan and cutting into 12 slices.

PER SERVING: Energy 190 calories; Protein 6 g; Carbohydrates 22 g; Dietary Fiber 3 g; Fat 9 g; Sugar 13 g; Cholesterol 30 mg; Sodium 50 mg

STORAGE
Refrigerator: **airtight container, 2 days**

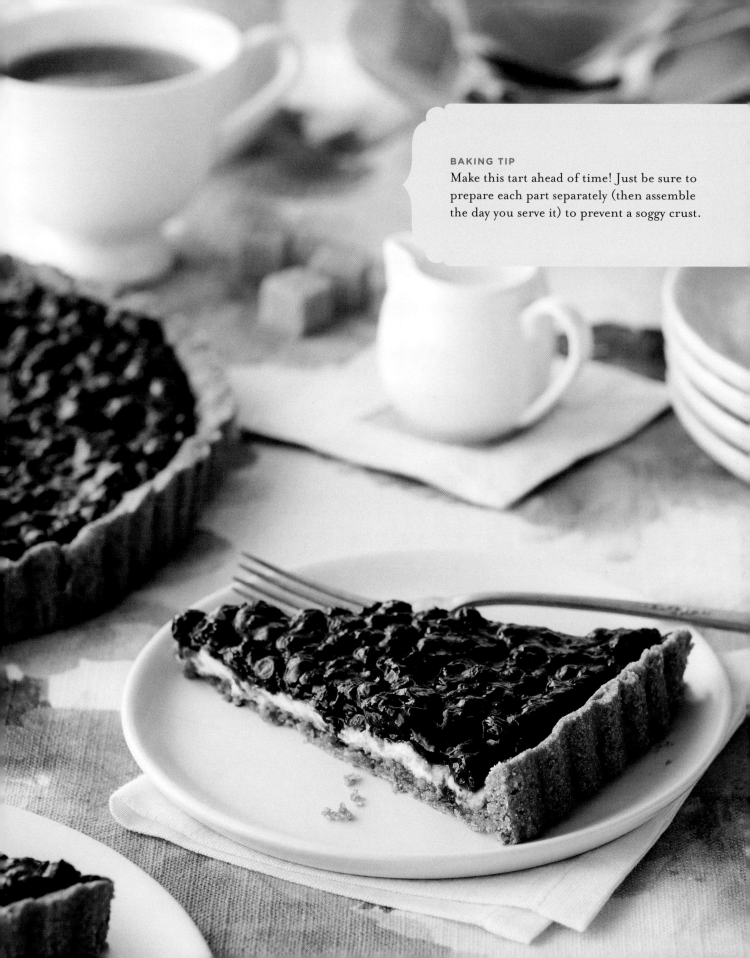

BAKING TIP
Make this tart ahead of time! Just be sure to prepare each part separately (then assemble the day you serve it) to prevent a soggy crust.

Carrot Spice Pie

A warm and spicy pie that tastes a lot like pumpkin pie, but is made with a
root vegetable most of us have in our refrigerators all the time: carrots!
Make this with Gluten-Free Pie Pastry I (page 102).

SERVES 8

1 recipe Gluten-Free Pie Pastry I
(page 102)

2 cups (500 mL) diced, cooked
carrots

¾ cup (175 mL) lightly packed
brown sugar

1 Tbsp (15 mL) arrowroot starch

½ tsp (2 mL) salt

2 tsp (10 mL) cinnamon

1 tsp (5 mL) ground ginger

½ tsp (2 mL) nutmeg

¼ tsp (1 mL) ground cloves

3 Tbsp (45 mL) orange juice

3 large eggs

1 ¼ cups (310 mL) 1% milk or
milk substitute

whipped cream (optional)

Prepare the Gluten-Free Pie Pastry I. Place it in a 9-inch
(23 cm) pie plate but don't bake it.

Preheat the oven to 425°F (220°C).

In a food processor or large blender, puree the carrots and
then add the sugar, starch, salt, cinnamon, ginger, nutmeg and
cloves. Blend. Add the orange juice, eggs and milk and blend
thoroughly. The mixture should be completely smooth. It is
extremely important to blend the filling thoroughly or it will
separate while baking. If you are unsure if it is blended enough,
pulse for another 2 to 4 minutes. Pour the mixture into the
prepared pastry shell.

Bake the pie for 12 minutes, then turn down the oven temperature
to 375°F (190°C). If the edges of the pastry appear to be browning
too quickly, cover them with strips of aluminum foil. Bake for 45 to
50 minutes, until the center of the pie is firm and the edges of the
crust are golden brown. Let cool completely and then chill in the
refrigerator for 1 to 2 hours. Best served cold. Top with whipped
cream (if using).

PER SERVING: Energy 120 calories; Protein 4 g; Carbohydrates 21 g;
Dietary Fiber 2 g; Fat 2.5 g; Sugar 17 g; Cholesterol 70 mg; Sodium 190 mg

STORAGE

Refrigerator: **airtight container or bag, 2–3 days**

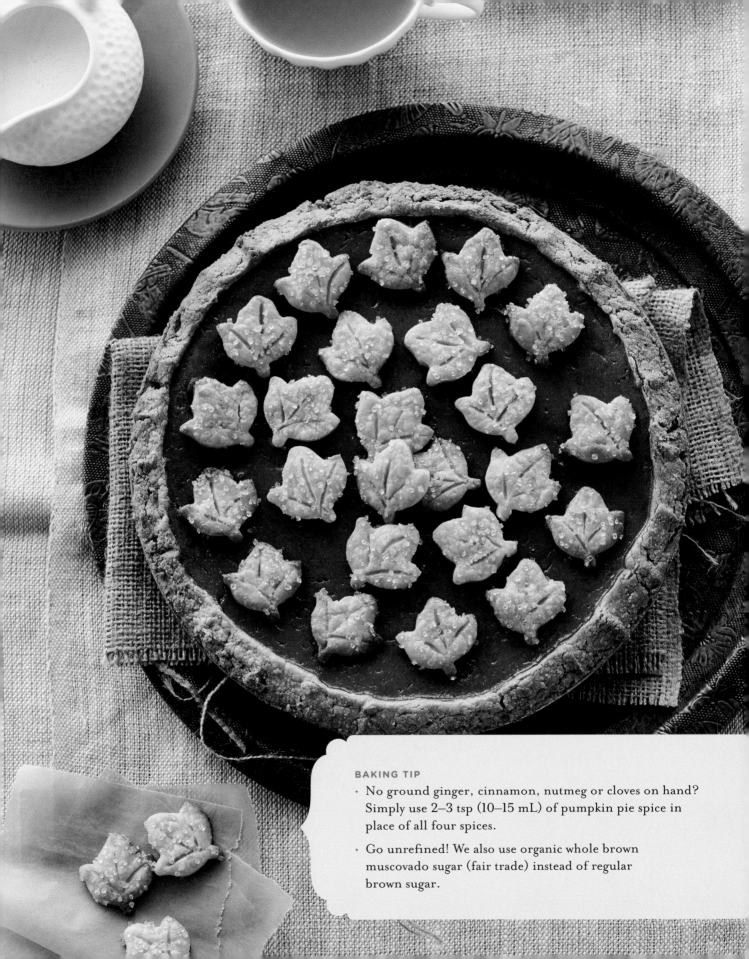

BAKING TIP

- No ground ginger, cinnamon, nutmeg or cloves on hand? Simply use 2–3 tsp (10–15 mL) of pumpkin pie spice in place of all four spices.

- Go unrefined! We also use organic whole brown muscovado sugar (fair trade) instead of regular brown sugar.

Pecan Date Pie

The added sweetness of dates gives this delicious, buttery pecan pie a unique twist.
Make this with Gluten-Free Pie Pastry II (page 103).

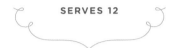

SERVES 12

1 recipe Gluten-Free
　　Pie Pastry II (page 103)

2 large eggs

½ cup (125 mL) unsalted butter,
　　melted and cooled

¾ cup (175 mL) lightly packed
　　brown sugar

¼ cup (60 mL) organic
　　cane sugar

1 Tbsp (15 mL) arrowroot
　　or potato starch

1 Tbsp (15 mL) whole (3.25%) milk
　　or milk substitute

1 tsp (5 mL) pure vanilla extract

1 cup (250 mL) chopped pecans

½ cup (125 mL) pitted, chopped
　　dates

Prepare the Gluten-Free Pie Pastry II. Use it to line a 9-inch (23 cm) pie plate.

Preheat the oven to 400°F (200°C).

In a large bowl, beat the eggs with a whisk until foamy. Stir in the melted butter, sugars and arrowroot starch. Mix well to combine. Stir in the milk and vanilla, then fold in the pecans and dates. Pour this into the unbaked crust.

Bake for 10 minutes. Turn down the oven temperature to 350°F (180°C). Bake for 30 to 35 minutes, until the top of the pie is firm and golden brown and the edges of the crust are also slightly golden brown. Allow it to cool for at least 30 minutes before serving. You can also serve this chilled if you prefer.

PER SERVING: Energy 330 calories; Protein 3 g; Carbohydrates 32 g; Dietary Fiber 3 g; Fat 20 g; Sugar 20 g; Cholesterol 70 mg; Sodium 70 mg

STORAGE
Refrigerator: **airtight container, 2–3 days**

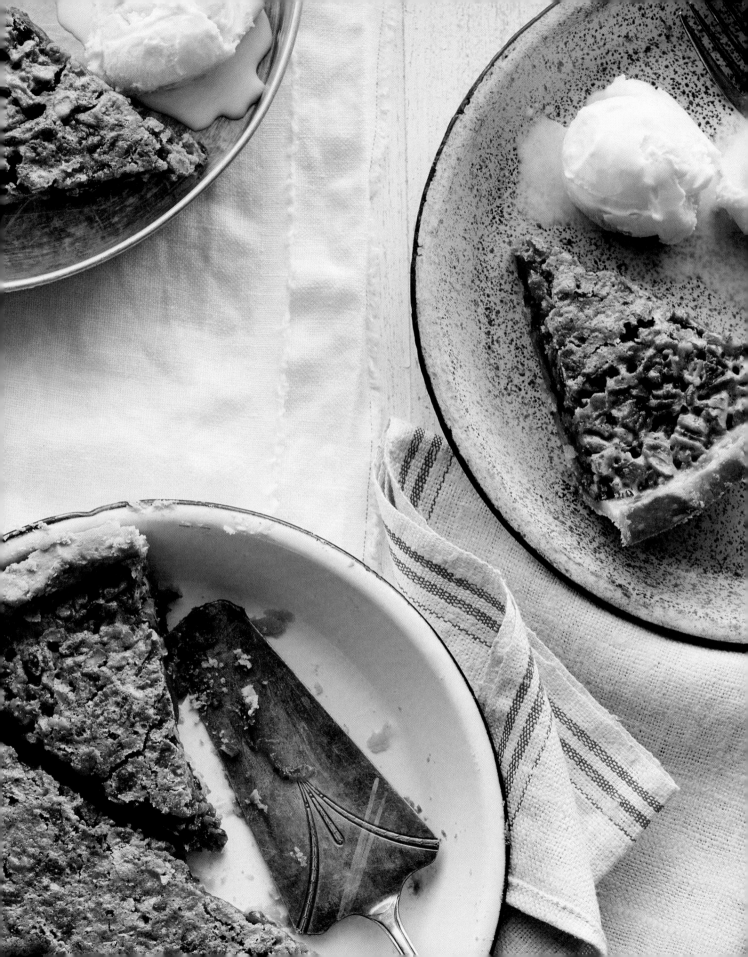

Chocolate Quinoa Pie

This pie has a thick and sweet chocolate filling made with cooked quinoa.
We use our Graham-Style Wafer Crumb Crust here, but Cream Cheese Pastry (page 104)
and Pressed Nut Crust (page 105) work equally well.

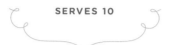

SERVES 10

Prepare the Graham-Style Wafer Crumb Crust and set aside.

Place the quinoa in a medium saucepan with 2 cups (500 mL) of water. Bring to a boil, turn down the heat to a simmer, cover and cook for 25 minutes. Fluff the quinoa with a fork, then let it sit, uncovered, to cool to room temperature.

In a food processor or large blender, puree the cooked quinoa with the milk, sugar, cocoa, maple syrup and vanilla. Puree repeatedly until the mixture is extremely smooth. If the mixture is too thick, use a spatula to adjust it in the blender and puree again. Pour the mixture into the prepared pastry shell.

Chill in the refrigerator, uncovered, until set, 1 to 2 hours. Best served cold with whipped cream (if using) and garnished with chocolate shavings (if using).

PER SERVING: Energy 220 calories; Protein 4 g; Carbohydrates 36 g; Dietary Fiber 3 g; Fat 7 g; Sugar 16 g; Cholesterol 15 mg; Sodium 50 mg

1 recipe Graham-Style Wafer Crumb Crust (page 108)

1 cup (250 mL) white or golden quinoa seeds

1 cup (250 mL) 1% or 2% milk or milk substitute

½ cup (125 mL) organic cane sugar

⅓ cup (75 mL) unsweetened cocoa powder

2 Tbsp (30 mL) pure maple syrup

1 tsp (5 mL) pure vanilla extract

whipped cream (optional)

chocolate shavings (optional)

BAKING TIP
Be sure not to cool the just-cooked quinoa in the refrigerator. Pureeing quinoa that is still warm or at least room temperature ensures that it gels together properly to make a nice thick pie.

STORAGE
Refrigerator: airtight container, 1-2 days

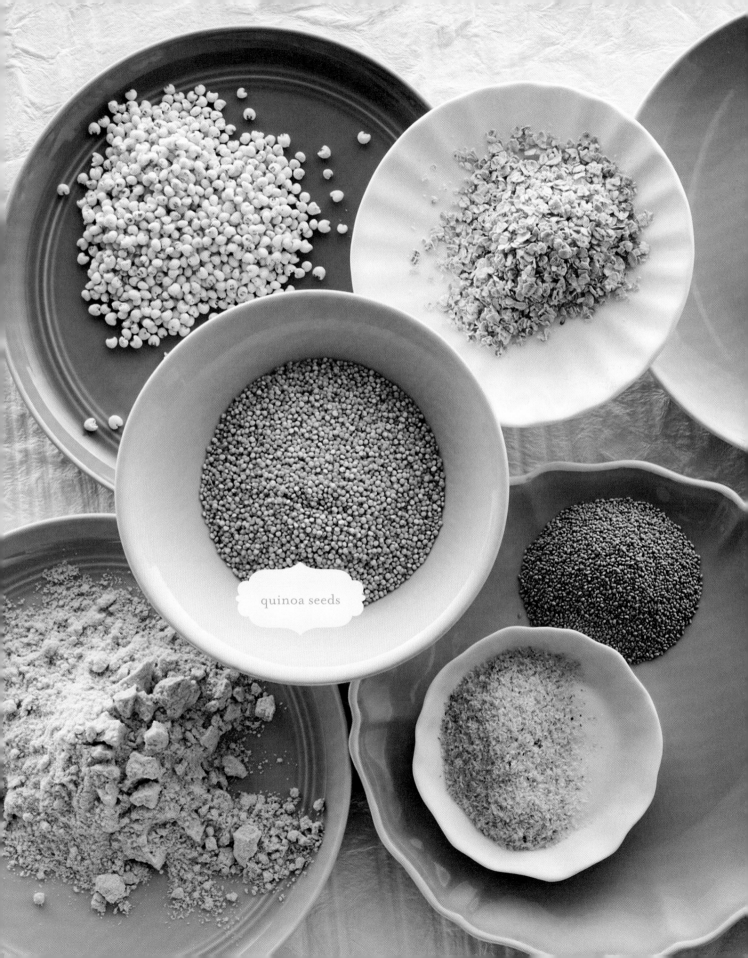

quinoa seeds

Tangy Lime Greek Yogurt Pie

Reminiscent of something you'd enjoy in a 50s-style diner, this cream pie has a sweet tangy lime flavor and a touch of coconut cream. It's all tucked inside a tasty graham crust made with our gluten-free Graham-Style Wafers (page 46) made from oat flour, oat bran and psyllium. This reinvented pie is truly swell.

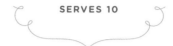

SERVES 10

TOPPING

½ cup (125 mL) chilled coconut milk (full fat) without emulsifiers (see note on facing page)

1 tsp (5 mL) organic cane sugar, pure maple syrup or desired sweetener

CRUST

1 ¼ cups (310 mL) crushed fine Graham-Style Wafers (page 46)

⅓ cup (75 mL) unsalted butter, melted

FILLING

11 oz (300 mL) can sweetened, condensed milk

½ cup (125 mL) fresh lime juice

3 Tbsp (45 mL) cornstarch

1 large egg

1 ½ cups (375 mL) 2% plain Greek yogurt

1 Tbsp (15 mL) lime zest

whipped cream for garnish

For the topping, ensure you open the coconut milk can from the top (that is, not the end it was standing on in the refrigerator). Pour off the coconut water into a jar to use for smoothies later (freeze it in an ice cube tray if desired). Scoop out the coconut cream from the can. It should be as thick as butter. Whip the coconut cream and sugar with a handheld or stand mixer until soft peaks form. Place the coconut cream in a large resealable plastic or piping bag and refrigerate for at least 2 hours.

Have a 9-inch (23 cm) pie plate ready. Preheat the oven to 325°F (160°C).

For the crust, mix the graham crumbs with the butter in a small bowl. Press it evenly into the pie plate and bake for 7 minutes. Remove from the oven and let cool completely. Set aside.

For the filling, place the condensed milk and lime juice in a medium saucepan. Bring to a simmer and allow to simmer for 5 minutes, or until it has reduced by about 25%. Set aside. Whisk the cornstarch and egg together in a medium bowl, then slowly whisk in the condensed milk mixture. Pour the contents of the bowl back into the saucepan and return to a full simmer on medium heat for 1 minute. Stir in the yogurt and lime zest.

Pour this mixture into the crust, cover with plastic wrap and chill in the refrigerator for at least 2 hours. Pipe whipped topping around the outside edges of the pie. Serve cold.

PER SERVING: Energy 450 calories; Protein 10 g; Carbohydrates 52 g; Dietary Fiber 2 g; Fat 19 g; Sugar 35 g; Cholesterol 60 mg; Sodium 150 mg

STORAGE

Refrigerator: **airtight container or bag, 4 days**

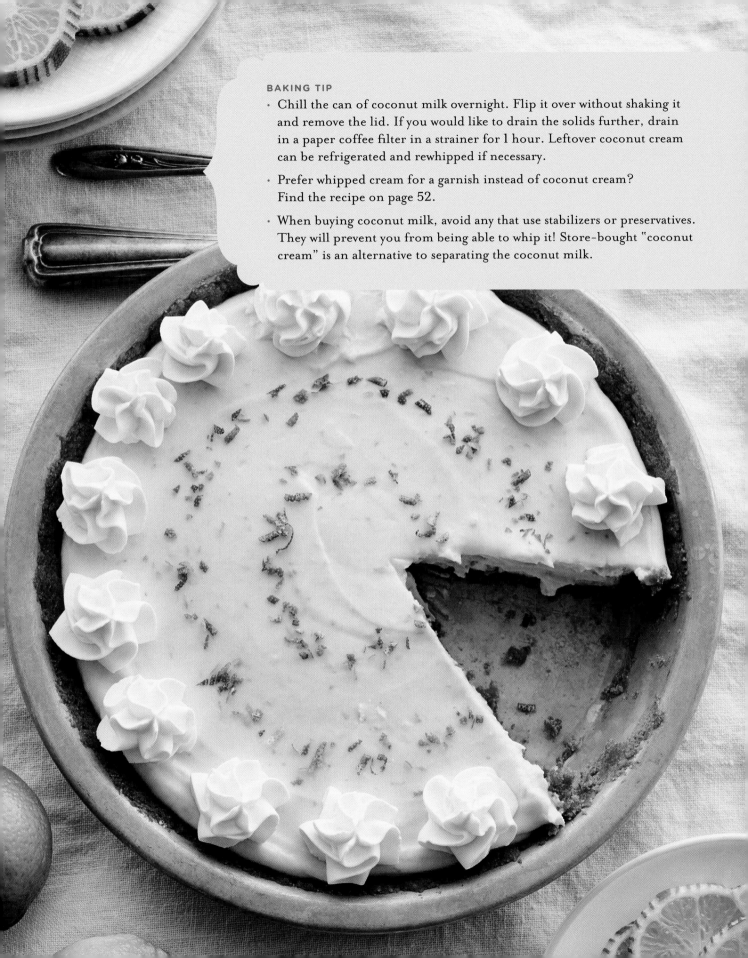

BAKING TIP

- Chill the can of coconut milk overnight. Flip it over without shaking it and remove the lid. If you would like to drain the solids further, drain in a paper coffee filter in a strainer for 1 hour. Leftover coconut cream can be refrigerated and rewhipped if necessary.

- Prefer whipped cream for a garnish instead of coconut cream? Find the recipe on page 52.

- When buying coconut milk, avoid any that use stabilizers or preservatives. They will prevent you from being able to whip it! Store-bought "coconut cream" is an alternative to separating the coconut milk.

Rich Chocolate Raspberry Tartlets

Pretty when posed on a platter, these tiny chocolate tarts made with sorghum, teff and a chocolate coconut filling are a brilliant finish to a brunch or dinner party. Prepare the tartlets and filling separately a few days in advance to easily throw together when you're ready to enjoy them. If you are really crunched for time, replace the ganache with chocolate hazelnut spread.

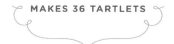

MAKES 36 TARTLETS

TARTLETS

⅓ cup (75 mL) teff flour

⅓ cup (75 mL) sorghum flour

3 Tbsp (45 mL) unsweetened cocoa powder

pinch salt

¼ cup (60 mL) liquid honey

3 Tbsp (45 mL) unsalted butter or virgin coconut oil, melted

GANACHE FILLING

14 oz (398 mL) can full-fat coconut milk, chilled, or ½ cup (125 mL) whipping cream, chilled

½ cup (125 mL) milk chocolate chips

36 fresh raspberries

Set aside two mini muffin tins. Preheat the oven to 325°F (160°C).

For the tartlets, place the teff and sorghum flours, cocoa and salt in a bowl and whisk together to combine. Work in the honey and butter with your hands until evenly mixed. Place 1 tsp (5 mL) of dough inside each muffin cup. Press into the bottom and use a wet finger to create a "cup" halfway up the sides. Bake in the oven for 8 minutes. Remove from the oven and press the bottoms down with a finger while still warm. Let cool completely.

For the filling, ensure you open the coconut milk can from the top (that is, not the end it was standing on in the refrigerator). Pour off the coconut water into a jar to use for smoothies later (freeze it in an ice cube tray if desired). Scoop out the coconut cream from the can. It should be as thick as butter. Heat ½ cup (125 mL) of the coconut cream to almost a simmer in a small saucepan. Remove from the heat and stir in the chocolate chips until completely melted. Let cool enough to touch, then pour 1 tsp (5 mL) of filling into each tartlet.

Chill the prepared tartlets for at least 30 minutes. Place a fresh raspberry on top of each one before serving.

PER SERVING: Energy 50 calories; Protein 1 g; Carbohydrates 5 g; Dietary Fiber 1 g; Fat 3.5 g; Sugar 2 g; Cholesterol 0 mg; Sodium 11 mg

STORAGE

Refrigerator: **airtight container, 2 days**

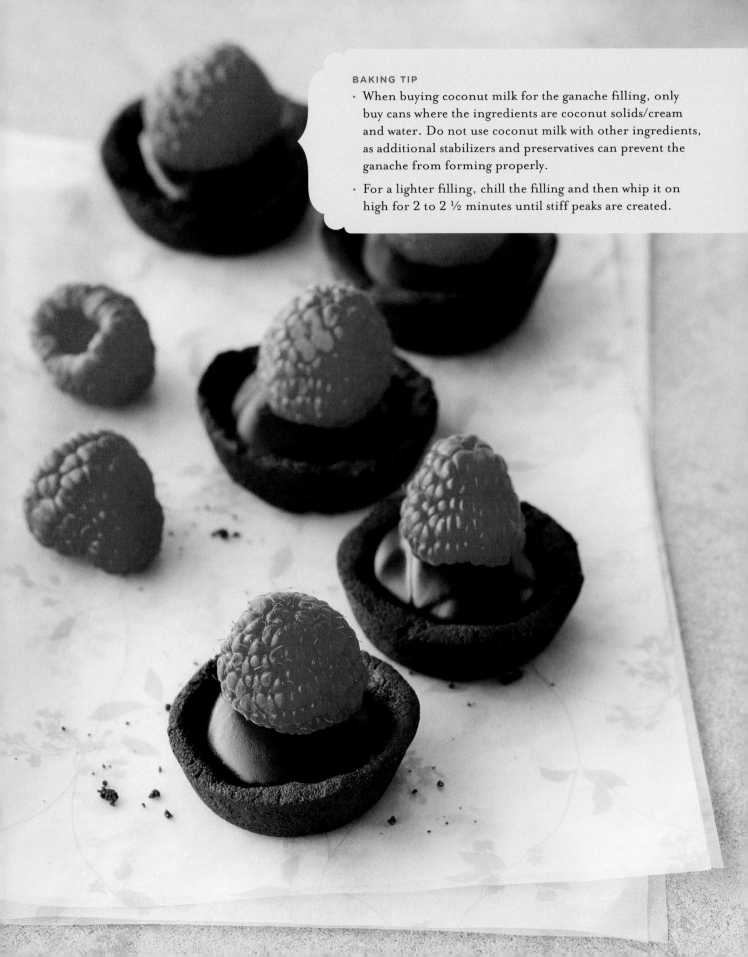

BAKING TIP

· When buying coconut milk for the ganache filling, only buy cans where the ingredients are coconut solids/cream and water. Do not use coconut milk with other ingredients, as additional stabilizers and preservatives can prevent the ganache from forming properly.

· For a lighter filling, chill the filling and then whip it on high for 2 to 2 ½ minutes until stiff peaks are created.

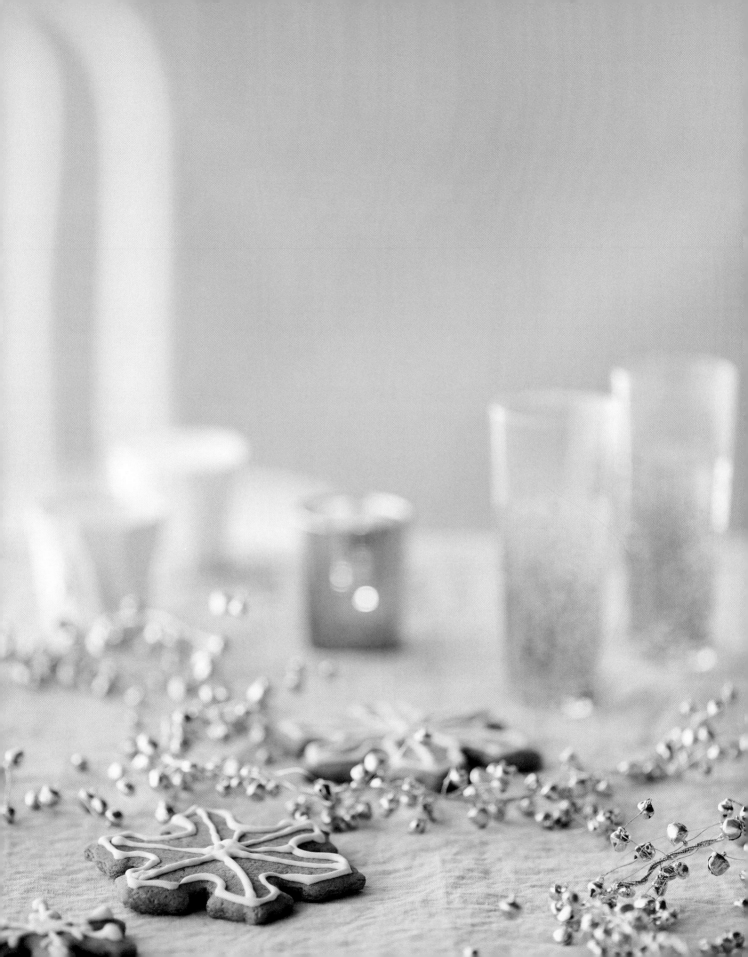

Special Occasion Baking

Yorkshire Pudding with Roasted Strawberries and Basil   133

Yogurt Cut-Out Cookies   134

Gingerbread Cookies   137

Double-Layer Chocolate Chia Zucchini Cake   138

Ancient Grain Summer Fruit Tarts   139

Honey-Roasted Beet and Lemon Cheesecake   140

Baked Apple Crumble with Carrot and Raisin Spice Filling   142

Sticky Toffee Pudding   144

Strawberry and Raspberry Coconut Cream Trifle   146

Teff-Crusted Ice Cream over Grilled Peaches
and Lavender Chamomile Syrup   149

Strawberry Shortcakes with Sweet Chantillly Cream   151

Thai Coconut Dark Chocolate Bark with Lime Zest   152

Candied Ginger, Orange and Pistachio Bark   153

Cherry Almond Truffles   154

Graham Peanut Butter Chocolate Bites   156

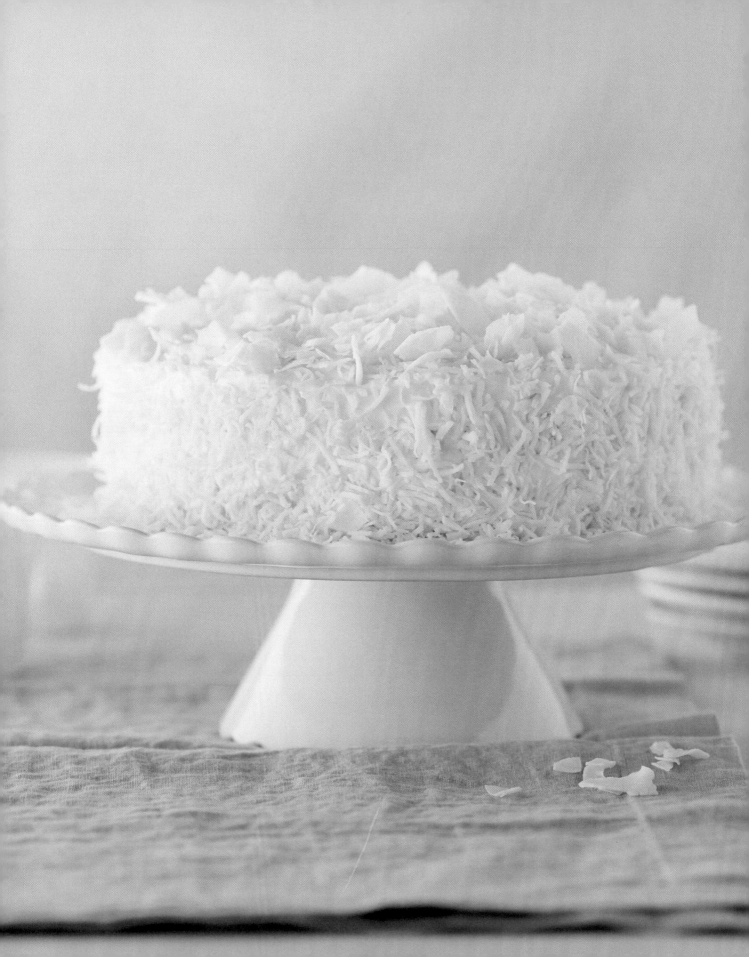

Holiday festivities and entertaining family and friends usually trigger the baking of an array of wonderful, tasty goodies that are satisfying, fun and all about pleasure. Bring people together, enjoy the moment and make memories with some revamped traditional favorites. Gluten-free ancient grains help to kick up the nutritional value while you indulge. For picnics or parties, whether you are surprising someone or involving loved ones in your baking process, you will find making the recipes in this chapter a gratifying experience that gets you in the mood to enjoy yourself and celebrate.

In need of a decadent celebration cake for an anniversary or maybe a birthday cake for the office? Try the Double-Layer Chocolate Chia Zucchini Cake (page 138) or the Honey-Roasted Beet and Lemon Cheesecake (page 140). Looking for something simple, sweet and unique? Try the quinoa- or millet-loaded Thai Coconut Dark Chocolate Bark with Lime Zest (page 152) or the Candied Ginger, Orange and Pistachio Bark (page 153). Need to bring a delicious dish to a gathering? Try Strawberry and Raspberry Coconut Cream Trifle (page 146) or the simple Cherry Almond Truffles (page 154). Also not to be missed are those classic favorites, now gluten-free, Gingerbread Cookies (page 137) and Yogurt Cut-Out Cookies (page 134).

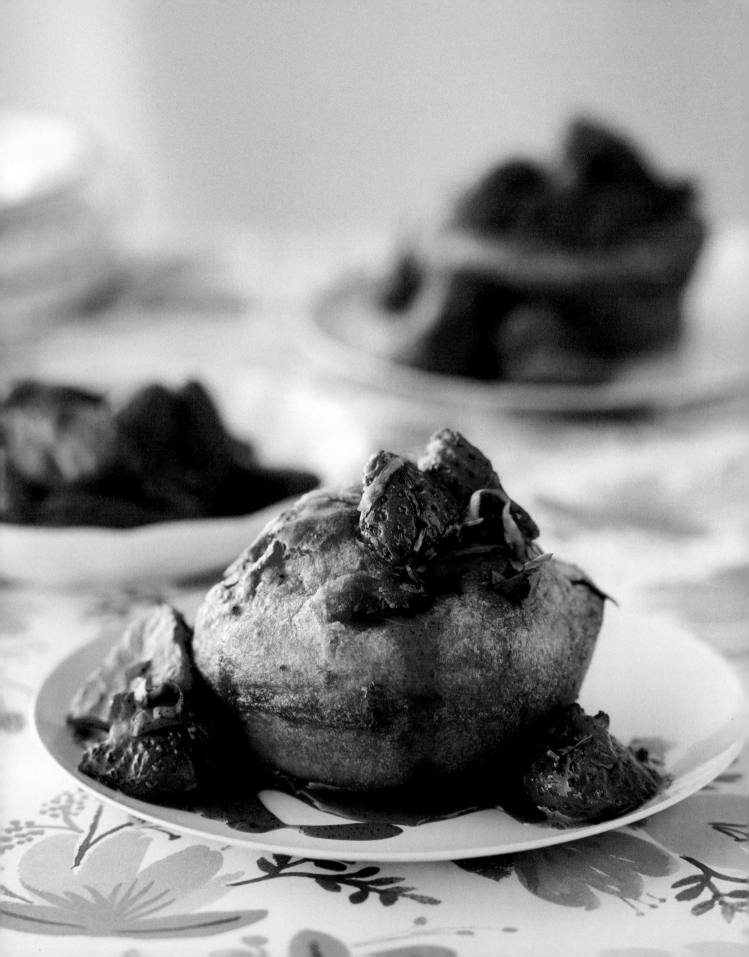

Yorkshire Pudding with Roasted Strawberries and Basil

Made with a combination of quinoa, sorghum and oat flours and tapioca starch, these warm and tender gluten–free Yorkshire puddings are light and chewy just as you'd expect them to be — but we've topped them with delicious roasted basil strawberries.

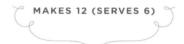

MAKES 12 (SERVES 6)

Preheat the oven to 425°F (220°C).

Scrape the seeds out of the vanilla bean and keep the pod. Toss the vanilla bean seeds and pod with the strawberries, basil and maple syrup in a 9-inch (2.5 L) square baking pan, stirring to evenly coat the strawberries. Bake for 15 minutes. Remove from the oven and set aside in the pan to cool. Discard the vanilla pod.

Generously spray or grease with cooking oil a 12-cup muffin pan. (This is essential for removing the puddings from the pan.) Turn down the oven temperature to 375°F (190°C).

Combine the quinoa, sorghum and oat flours with the tapioca starch in a medium bowl. Set aside.

In a separate medium bowl, beat the eggs and milk. Stir into the flour mixture and set aside. Divide the butter evenly among the muffin cups, about ½ tsp (2.5 mL) for each. Place the pan in the oven to melt the butter, 2 to 5 minutes. Remove the pan from the oven and distribute the batter evenly among the muffin cups.

Bake for 5 minutes. Turn down the oven temperature to 350°F (180°C) and bake for 30 to 32 minutes, until the tops are puffed and golden. Scatter roasted strawberries overtop and serve warm.

Eat these the day you make them.

PER SERVING: Energy 200 calories; Protein 7 g; Carbohydrates 25 g; Dietary Fiber 3 g; Fat 8 g; Sugar 9 g; Cholesterol 105 mg; Sodium 60 mg

1 vanilla bean

2 cups (500 mL) fresh or frozen, hulled and sliced strawberries

2 Tbsp (30 mL) chopped fresh basil

2 Tbsp (30 mL) pure maple syrup

¼ cup (60 mL) quinoa flour

¼ cup (60 mL) sorghum flour

¼ cup (60 mL) oat flour

¼ cup (60 mL) tapioca starch

3 large eggs

1 cup (250 mL) 2% milk

2 Tbsp (30 mL) unsalted butter

BAKING TIP
When grinding your whole oats into oat flour, ensure you grind until you obtain the finest consistency possible. This will ensure there are no coarse bits in your fluffy Yorkshire puddings!

Yogurt Cut-Out Cookies

No matter the occasion, all you need to do is decide how you are going to decorate these cookies. Ancient grain goodness is hiding in the sweet sorghum flour, but you can glam up these gems using traditional sprinkles, candies or icing. Make your own dye-free decorating sugar or icing by following the tip on the facing page.

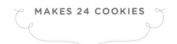

MAKES 24 COOKIES

1 cup (250 mL) sorghum flour

1 cup (250 mL) tapioca starch, plus extra for dusting

½ tsp (2 mL) xanthan gum

1 tsp (5 mL) baking powder

¼ tsp (1 mL) baking soda

½ tsp (2 mL) salt

⅔ cup (150 mL) unsalted butter

1 ¼ cups (310 mL) ground Sucanat or organic cane sugar

½ cup (125 mL) 1% or 2% plain yogurt

2 large eggs

2 tsp (10 mL) pure vanilla extract

1 tsp (5 mL) almond extract

Line a large baking sheet with parchment paper.

Place the sorghum flour, tapioca starch, xanthan gum, baking powder, baking soda and salt in a medium bowl and whisk to combine. Set aside.

In a separate large bowl, beat the butter with the sugar until smooth, then add the yogurt, eggs, vanilla extract and almond extract and mix well. Gradually add the flour mixture, stirring until fully incorporated. Chill the dough for 2 hours.

Preheat the oven to 350°F (180°C).

Remove the dough from the fridge and use your hands to work it for a few moments so that it's ready to roll. Roll out to ⅛ inch (0.3 cm) thickness using tapioca starch for dusting. Use a 2 ½-inch (6 cm) cookie cutter to cut out the dough and place on the baking sheet 1 inch (2.5 cm) apart.

Bake for 10 to 12 minutes, until the edges are slightly golden. Let cool completely on the baking sheet, then transfer to a wire rack to decorate as desired.

PER SERVING: Energy 150 calories; Protein 2 g; Carbohydrates 24 g; Dietary Fiber 1 g; Fat 6 g; Sugar 10 g; Cholesterol 20 mg; Sodium 80 mg

STORAGE

Room Temperature: **airtight container or bag, 7 days**

Refrigerator: **airtight container or bag, 7 days**

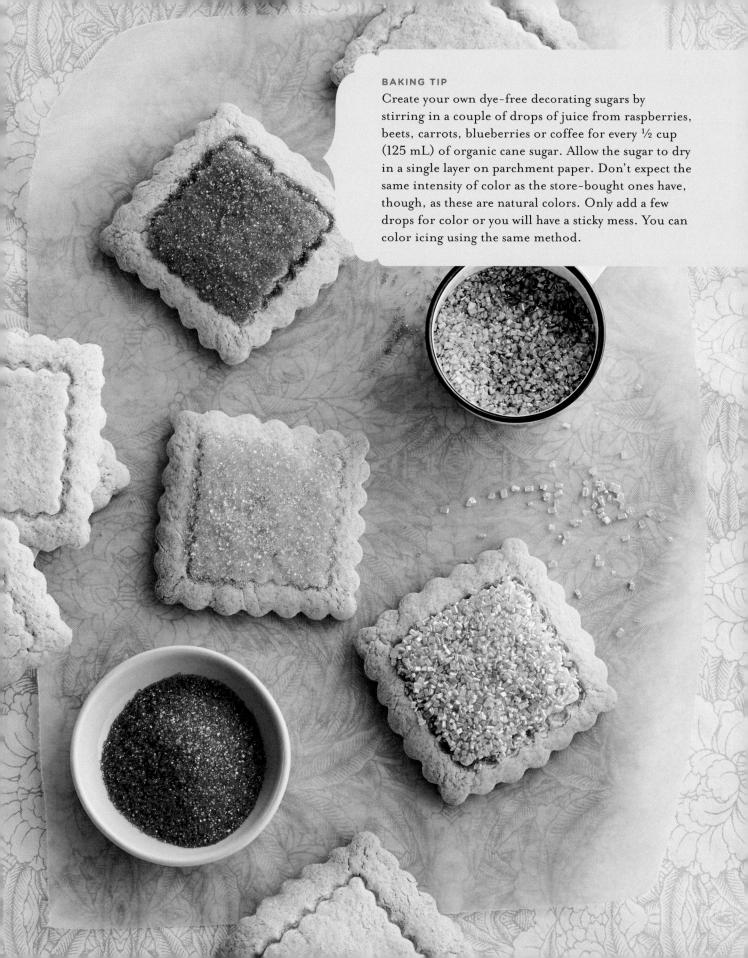

BAKING TIP
Create your own dye-free decorating sugars by stirring in a couple of drops of juice from raspberries, beets, carrots, blueberries or coffee for every ½ cup (125 mL) of organic cane sugar. Allow the sugar to dry in a single layer on parchment paper. Don't expect the same intensity of color as the store-bought ones have, though, as these are natural colors. Only add a few drops for color or you will have a sticky mess. You can color icing using the same method.

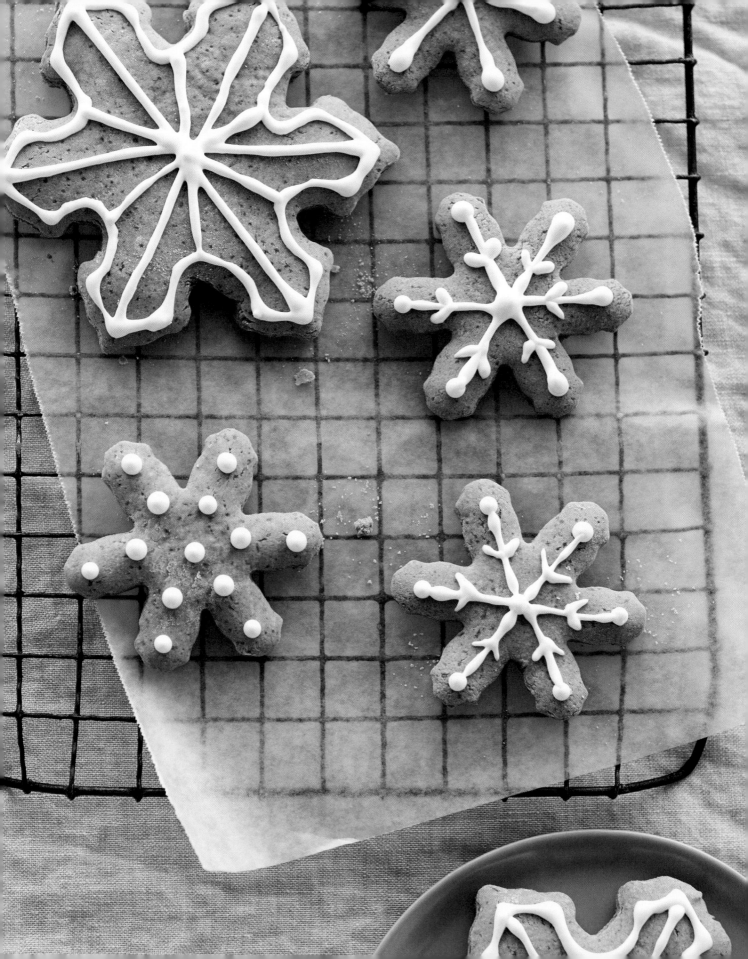

Gingerbread Cookies

Whatever their shape or design, the sweet ginger and molasses smell of gingerbread cookies baking in the oven is noticeably wonderful (not to mention, usually complete with memories!) when it fills the house. Decorate this version, made with sorghum and oats, with your own touch of sparkle and color. This light–colored gingerbread is ideal for a variety of holiday decorations.

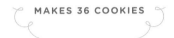

MAKES 36 COOKIES

Line a large baking sheet with parchment paper.

Place the sorghum and oat flours, tapioca starch, xanthan gum, ginger, cinnamon, baking soda and salt in a medium bowl and whisk to combine. Set aside.

In a large bowl or a stand mixer, mix the butter, sugar, molasses and egg until smooth. Gradually add the flour mixture until a dough is formed. Divide the dough in half and form two disks. Wrap each one with plastic wrap and chill for 2 hours.

Preheat the oven to 350°F (180°C).

Roll the dough out on a lightly floured surface to ⅛ inch (0.3 cm) thickness. Use a 2-inch (5 cm) cookie cutter (or your preferred shape) to cut out the cookies and place them on the prepared baking sheet 1 inch (2.5 cm) apart. Repeat with the remaining dough. Bake the cookies until the edges are starting to turn a slight golden brown, 8 to 10 minutes. Let the cookies cool completely on a rack before decorating.

PER SERVING: Energy 110 calories; Protein 2 g; Carbohydrates 16 g; Dietary Fiber 1 g; Fat 4 g; Sugar 5 g; Cholesterol 20 mg; Sodium 80 mg

1 cup (250 mL) sorghum flour

⅔ cup (150 mL) oat flour

1 cup (250 mL) tapioca starch, plus some for dusting

¾ tsp (3 mL) xanthan gum

1 Tbsp (15 mL) ground ginger

1 ½ tsp (7 mL) cinnamon

1 tsp (5 mL) baking soda

¼ tsp (1 mL) salt

⅔ cup (150 mL) unsalted butter, softened

½ cup (125 mL) ground Sucanat or organic cane sugar

2 Tbsp (30 mL) molasses

1 large egg

STORAGE

Room Temperature: **airtight container or bag, 7 days**

Refrigerator: **airtight container or bag, 7 days**

Double-Layer Chocolate Chia Zucchini Cake

Millet, oat, sorghum and chia along with zucchini are in this fabulous gluten-free, moist double-layer chocolate cake! And not only is it delicious, it also makes a beautiful decorated cake for any occasion. Try it with the frosting from the Outrageous Quinoa Chocolate Cake (page 91).

MAKES ONE DOUBLE-LAYER 8-INCH (1.2 L) ROUND OR 9-INCH (2 L) SQUARE CAKE (SERVES 12) OR 12 LARGE CUPCAKES

1 Tbsp (15 mL) ground chia seeds

¼ cup (60 mL) boiling water

⅓ cup (75 mL) millet flour

⅓ cup (75 mL) oat flour

⅓ cup (75 mL) sorghum flour

½ cup (125 mL) unsweetened cocoa powder

½ tsp (2 mL) baking soda

½ tsp (2 mL) baking powder

¼ cup (60 mL) unsalted butter, softened

¾ cup (175 mL) lightly packed brown sugar

2 large eggs

1 tsp (5 mL) pure vanilla extract

1 cup (250 mL) grated zucchini, packed

Lightly grease two 8-inch (1.2 L) round or 9-inch (2 L) square baking pans. Line the bottom of each pan with parchment paper. Preheat the oven to 350°F (180°C).

Place the chia in a small bowl with the boiling water. Gently stir with a fork to ensure the ground seeds are evenly distributed. Set aside to thicken, about 10 minutes.

In a medium bowl, combine the millet, oat and sorghum flours, cocoa, baking soda and baking powder.

In a separate bowl, cream the butter with the sugar and the chia mixture. Add the eggs one at a time, followed by the vanilla, and mix well. Stir the butter mixture into the flour mixture until just mixed. Add the zucchini and stir until just blended. Pour the batter evenly into the two pans.

Bake for 17 to 18 minutes (20 minutes for cupcakes), until the middle springs back when gently pressed or a toothpick inserted in the center comes out with only a few small crumbs. Let cool in the pan. If frosting, refrigerate for 2 hours first.

PER SERVING: Energy 140 calories; Protein 3 g; Carbohydrates 19 g; Dietary Fiber 2 g; Fat 6 g; Sugar 9 g; Cholesterol 40 mg; Sodium 70 mg

BAKING TIP
Shred the zucchini before you start your recipe and let it sit for about 10 minutes in a sieve to drain off excess water before using.

STORAGE
Refrigerator: airtight container, 1-2 days

Ancient Grain Summer Fruit Tarts

These individual, flat tarts are made from oat, quinoa and sorghum ancient grain flours and have a light layer of sweetened cream cheese topped with juicy and colorful sliced fruit for a pretty presentation.

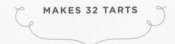

MAKES 32 TARTS

Place paper muffin cup liners in three 12-cup muffin pans. Pour some water into the 4 empty cups to avoid burning them. Preheat the oven to 350°F (180°C).

For the tarts, place the oat, quinoa and sorghum flours, tapioca starch, baking powder and salt in a large bowl and whisk to combine. Set aside.

Place the coconut oil, brown sugar, egg, milk, vanilla extract and almond extract in a medium bowl and mix well. Add the coconut oil mixture to the flour mixture and stir just enough to combine. Using a tablespoon or 1 ½-inch (4 cm) scoop, place a ball of dough into the bottom of each muffin cup and press down to flatten completely.

Bake for 8 to 10 minutes, until the edges and tops are slightly golden. Keeping the pastry in the paper liners, remove from the muffin pans and transfer to a rack to cool completely. (If you don't have three muffin tins you can bake these in batches. Just be sure to let the pans cool before you add more dough.)

For the topping, mix the cream cheese and maple syrup with a handheld mixer or rotary beater until fluffy. Remove the paper liners from the tarts when completely cooled and spread the base of each tart evenly with 1 ½ to 2 teaspoons (7–10 mL) of cream cheese mixture. Place some chopped fruit on top of the cream cheese. Serve immediately or allow to cool in the refrigerator for up to 1 hour.

PER SERVING: Energy 120 calories; Protein 1 g; Carbohydrates 10 g; Dietary Fiber 1 g; Fat 8 g; Sugar 5 g; Cholesterol 15 mg; Sodium 45 mg

TARTS

⅔ cup (150 mL) oat flour

½ cup (125 mL) quinoa flour

⅓ cup (75 mL) sorghum flour

¼ cup (60 mL) tapioca starch

1 tsp (5 mL) baking powder

¼ tsp (1 mL) salt

¾ cup (175 mL) virgin coconut oil

½ cup (125 mL) lightly packed brown sugar

1 large egg

1 Tbsp (15 mL) 1% or 2% milk or milk substitute

½ tsp (2 mL) pure vanilla extract

½ tsp (2 mL) pure almond extract

TOPPING

8 oz (225 g) package plain cream cheese, softened

¼ cup (60 mL) pure maple syrup or powdered (icing) sugar

½ cup (125 mL) peeled and sliced fresh kiwi

½ cup (125 mL) sliced fresh strawberries

½ cup (125 mL) chopped fresh apples

½ cup (125 mL) chopped fresh pineapple

STORAGE

Refrigerator: **airtight container, 2 days**

Honey-Roasted Beet and Lemon Cheesecake

Yogurt cheese makes this cheesecake with fewer calories than the traditional cream cheese version! Using the Graham–Style Wafer Crumb Crust (page 108) means you can make this beauty completely gluten–free. Roasted beets with honey and lemon provide the perfect sweet topping with a shot of nutrition! This is superb for entertaining or when you want to bake something that is a showstopper! Make the yogurt cheese two days before and the cheesecake one day before you plan to serve it so it has time to chill.

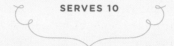

SERVES 10

4 cups (1 L) plain 2% gelatin-free yogurt

1–2 medium whole beets (enough to yield 1 ½ cups/375 mL peeled, chopped beets)

⅓ cup + 3 Tbsp (120 mL) liquid honey

1 Tbsp (15 mL) grapeseed oil

3 tsp (15 mL) fresh lemon juice, divided

1 Tbsp + 1 tsp (20 mL) lemon zest

3 large eggs, beaten

1 Tbsp (15 mL) cornstarch

2 tsp (10 mL) pure vanilla extract

1 baked, 10-inch (3 L) Graham–Style Wafer Crumb Crust (page 108) in a springform pan

2 Tbsp (30 mL) water

2 tsp (10 mL) cornstarch

Line a large sieve with one or two paper towels and place it over a medium bowl. Place the yogurt inside the strainer and allow it to sit overnight in the refrigerator.

The following day, preheat the oven to 375°F (180°C).

Ensure the greens are removed from the beets and place the whole, washed beets in a parchment bag or on one half of a large piece of aluminum foil on a large baking sheet. Drizzle with 3 Tbsp (45 mL) of honey, grapeseed oil, 2 tsp (10 mL) of lemon juice and 1 tsp (5 mL) of lemon zest. Seal the parchment bag by folding the opening over a few times or fold the aluminum foil over to seal.

Bake for 25 to 35 minutes, until the beets are fork-tender. Set aside and allow to cool. When cooled, gently rub the beets with your fingers to remove the outer skins and cut them into large chunks. Discard the skins.

STORAGE

Refrigerator: **airtight container, 3-4 days**

Turn down the oven temperature to 325°F (160°C).

The yogurt should now have drained and thickened, making yogurt cheese. Discard the liquid from the yogurt and place the firmed and thickened yogurt cheese in a large bowl. Add the remaining ⅓ cup (75 mL) of honey, eggs, cornstarch, vanilla, remaining 1 tsp (5 mL) of lemon juice and remaining 1 Tbsp (15 mL) of lemon zest. Beat the mixture using a rotary handheld beater, handheld mixer or immersion blender until well blended.

Scoop the cheesecake mixture into the prepared (and cooled) graham crust in the springform pan. Bake for 45 to 50 minutes, until the cheesecake is firm to touch in the middle and the edges are lightly golden and beginning to pull away from the edges of the pan. Remove from the oven and allow to cool in the pan.

Meanwhile, in a medium saucepan, puree the beets in 2 Tbsp (30 mL) of water with a handheld mixer or immersion blender, taking care not to splash yourself with beet juice. Set over high heat and add the cornstarch. (**NOTE**: You may need to add some water, depending on how much water your beets have retained.) Bring to a boil. Turn down the heat to a simmer and cook, stirring constantly, until the mixture thickens slightly, about 10 minutes. (**NOTE**: Depending on how naturally sweet or bitter your beets are, you may wish to add some additional honey to taste.)

Allow the sauce to cool. When both the sauce and the cheesecake have cooled completely, chill them in the refrigerator for at least 1 hour before serving. Slice the cheesecake and top with honey-roasted beet sauce to serve.

PER SERVING: Energy 260 calories; Protein 7 g; Carbohydrates 37 g; Dietary Fiber 2 g; Fat 10 g; Sugar 23 g; Cholesterol 75 mg; Sodium 140 mg

BAKING TIP
· Top this cheesecake with chocolate, blackberry or strawberry sauce, or any of your favorite cheesecake toppings!

· No gelatin! Yogurt will likely be clearly labeled if it does not contain gelatin. However, if it is not obvious, simply ensure it is not on the product's list of ingredients. Yogurt that contains gelatin will not allow retained water to drain off.

Baked Apple Crumble with Carrot and Raisin Spice Filling

The warm flavors of cinnamon and cloves in this baked apple crumble combine with the oats, carrot, millet and brown sugar to make this a perfect treat. It's especially tasty with a small side of ice cream.

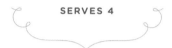

SERVES 4

4 Empire or Gala apples, skin on, cored almost to bottom

FILLING

⅓ cup (75 mL) grated carrot

6 tsp (90 mL) lightly packed brown sugar

3 Tbsp (45 mL) seedless raisins

½ tsp (2 mL) cinnamon

½ tsp (2 mL) lemon zest

pinch ground cloves

TOPPING

¼ cup (60 mL) old-fashioned rolled oats

1 Tbsp (15 mL) millet, sorghum or quinoa flour

1 Tbsp (15 mL) lightly packed brown sugar

1 Tbsp (15 mL) unsalted butter, softened

pinch cinnamon

pinch salt (optional)

Have a 9-inch (2 L) or 13- × 9-inch (3.5 L) baking pan ready. Preheat the oven to 375°F (190°C).

Use a knife to slice a shallow line around the circumference of each apple (this will prevent the apple from splitting when it bakes). Cut a thin slice off the bottom of each apple so they can stand securely in the baking dish.

For the filling, place the carrot, sugar, raisins, cinnamon, lemon zest and cloves in a small bowl and mix to combine. Set aside.

For the topping, in a separate small bowl, use your hands to mix together the oats, millet flour, brown sugar, butter, cinnamon and salt (if using) until the butter is incorporated and the mixture looks like pea-sized crumbs. Set aside.

Fill the center of each apple with filling. Divide the topping among the apples (if some of it falls into the dish, that is okay). Cover the pan loosely with foil and bake for 45 minutes, or until the apples are tender. Serve with ice cream, if desired.

PER SERVING: Energy 220 calories; Protein 2 g; Carbohydrates 45 g; Dietary Fiber 4 g; Fat 3.5 g; Sugar 21 g; Cholesterol 10 mg; Sodium 15 mg

STORAGE

Refrigerator: **airtight container, 3 days**

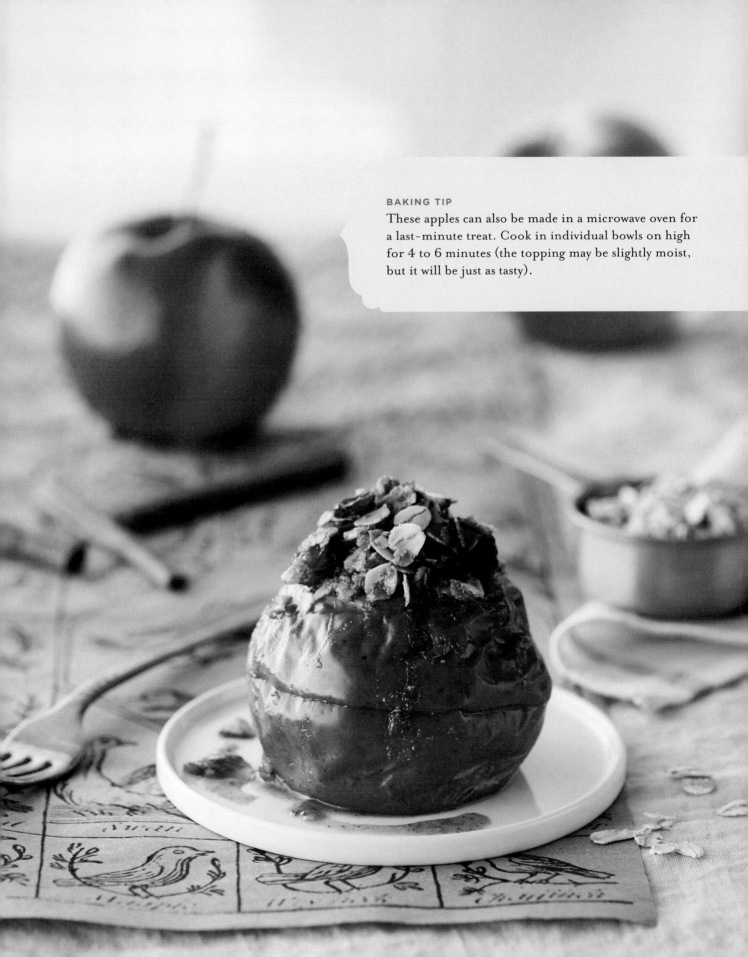

BAKING TIP

These apples can also be made in a microwave oven for a last-minute treat. Cook in individual bowls on high for 4 to 6 minutes (the topping may be slightly moist, but it will be just as tasty).

Sticky Toffee Pudding

This decadent, moist cake drizzled with sweet, soft caramel is a common family favorite often served during popular holidays.

SERVES 16

CAKE

2 cups (500 mL) pitted, chopped dates

1 Tbsp (15 mL) ground chia seeds

1 cup (250 mL) boiling water

¾ cup (175 mL) oat flour

⅓ cup (75 mL) sorghum flour

⅓ cup (75 mL) millet flour

⅓ cup (75 mL) arrowroot starch

2 tsp (10 mL) baking powder

1 tsp (5 mL) baking soda

½ cup (125 mL) lightly packed brown sugar

¼ cup (60 mL) unsalted butter, softened

¼ cup (60 mL) 1% plain yogurt

2 large eggs

2 Tbsp (30 mL) pure maple syrup

1 tsp (5 mL) pure vanilla extract

½ cup (125 mL) chopped walnuts (toasted if you prefer)

CARAMEL

¾ cup (175 mL) 18% cream

1 cup (250 mL) lightly packed brown sugar

⅓ cup (75 mL) unsalted butter

Lightly spray with cooking oil or grease a 9-inch (2.5 L) square baking pan. Line the pan with parchment paper. Preheat the oven to 350°F (180°C).

For the cake, place the dates and chia in a medium bowl with the boiling water. Gently stir with a fork to ensure everything is evenly distributed. Set aside to thicken the chia and hydrate the dates, 5 to 10 minutes.

In a separate large bowl, use a whisk to combine the oat, sorghum and millet flours, arrowroot starch, baking powder and baking soda. Mix well and set aside.

In a separate medium bowl, mix together the brown sugar, softened butter, yogurt, eggs, maple syrup and vanilla. Beat well. Add the butter mixture to the flour mixture and continue to mix until combined. Fold in the date mixture with its soaking liquid. Pour the mixture into the prepared pan and bake for 30 to 35 minutes, until a toothpick inserted in the center comes out clean.

For the caramel, in a medium saucepan over high heat, mix the cream with the brown sugar and butter. Bring to a boil. Turn down the heat to a simmer and cook, stirring constantly, until the mixture thickens slightly, about 10 minutes.

Remove the cake from the oven and pour the caramel sauce overtop while it's still warm and in the pan. Sprinkle with the walnuts. Serve warm.

PER SERVING: Energy 300 calories; Protein 4 g; Carbohydrates 43 g; Dietary Fiber 3 g; Fat 13 g; Sugar 27 g; Cholesterol 55 mg; Sodium 100 mg

STORAGE

Refrigerator: **airtight container, 1-2 days**

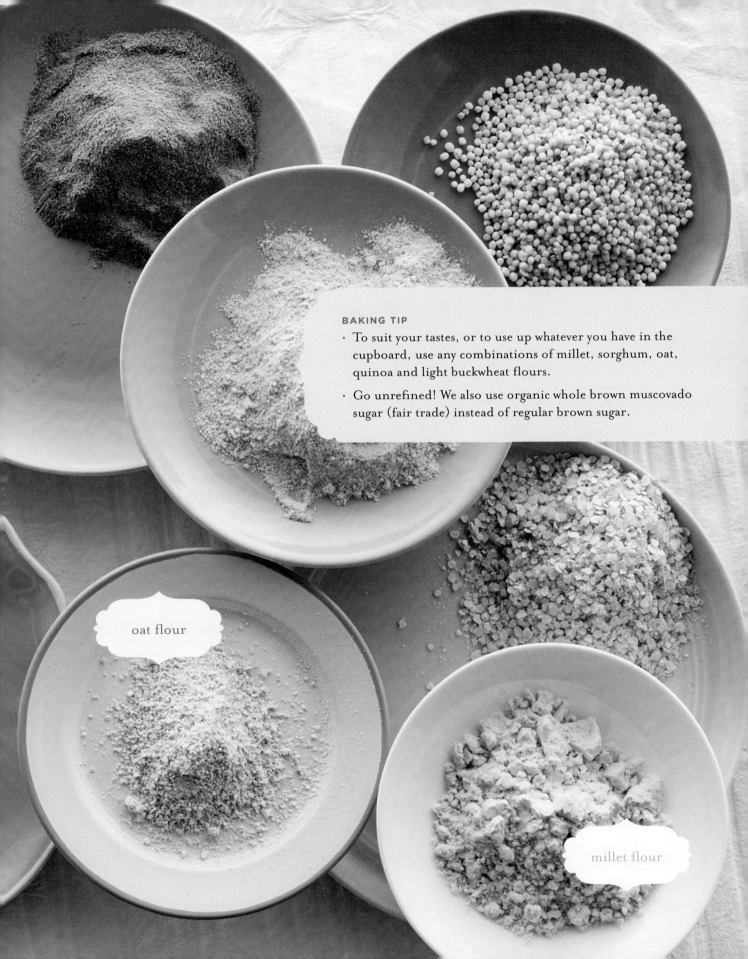

BAKING TIP

· To suit your tastes, or to use up whatever you have in the cupboard, use any combinations of millet, sorghum, oat, quinoa and light buckwheat flours.

· Go unrefined! We also use organic whole brown muscovado sugar (fair trade) instead of regular brown sugar.

oat flour

millet flour

Strawberry and Raspberry Coconut Cream Trifle

The Ancient Grain Pound Cake (page 80) comes to life in this fruit- and cream-filled favorite. Coconut milk and whipped cream combined with fresh raspberries and strawberries make a luxurious and gluten-free treat.

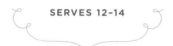

SERVES 12-14

1 Ancient Grain Pound Cake (page 80)

2 cans (14 oz/398 mL each) light coconut milk

½ cup (125 mL) organic cane sugar

¼ cup (60 mL) cornstarch

2 tsp (10 mL) pure vanilla extract

3 ½ cups (875 mL) reduced-fat whipping cream

¼ cup (60 mL) powdered (icing) sugar

3 cups (750 mL) fresh strawberries, sliced

3 cups (750 mL) fresh raspberries

Cut the Ancient Grain Pound Cake into ½-inch (1 cm) pieces (you want them bite-sized) and set aside.

In a large saucepan, bring the coconut milk, sugar and cornstarch to a boil over medium heat, stirring constantly. Turn down the heat and continue to cook at a simmer for 5 minutes. Stir in the vanilla and remove from the heat. Allow to cool slightly, then cover and chill in the refrigerator for 2 hours.

Beat the whipping cream with the powdered sugar until thick. Fold the whipped cream into the chilled coconut mixture and set aside.

In a 9-inch (2 L) clear serving dish or bowl, place half of the coconut cream in the bottom, followed by a layer of half of the cake chunks. Top with half of the strawberries and raspberries. Place the remaining half of the cake chunks on top of the fruit layer, followed by another layer of coconut cream (reserving 1 cup/250 mL of coconut cream) and then the remaining fruit. Top with the reserved 1 cup (250 mL) of coconut cream. Chill for an hour or more before serving. This can be made the night before you plan to eat it.

PER SERVING: Energy 410 calories; Protein 4 g; Carbohydrates 35 g; Dietary Fiber 3 g; Fat 23 g; Sugar 19 g; Cholesterol 97 mg; Sodium 82 mg

STORAGE

Refrigerator: **airtight container, 1-2 days**

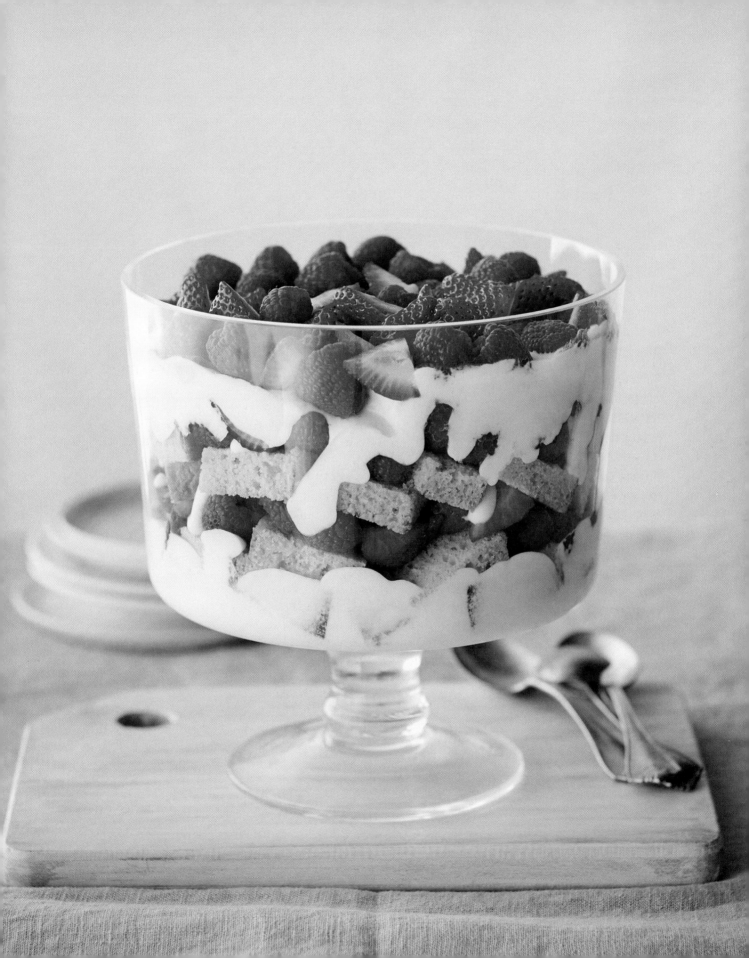

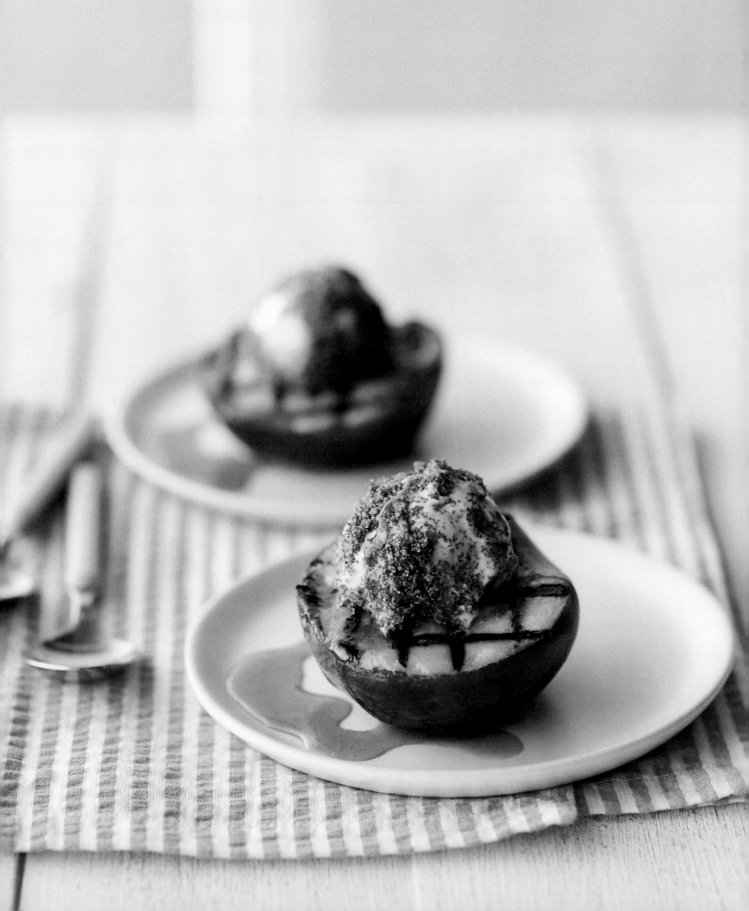

Teff-Crusted Ice Cream over Grilled Peaches and Lavender Chamomile Syrup

Looking for something elegant and out of the ordinary that will leave your taste buds singing an operatic score? Teff! The fusion of flavors in grilled peaches drizzled with warm lavender chamomile syrup and topped with ice cream (yes, cold ice cream) encrusted with the slight crunch of sweetened, toasted teff will be a pleasant surprise.

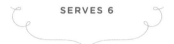

SERVES 6

Cut a large piece of parchment and set it aside.

For the ice cream balls, melt the butter with the brown sugar in a small saucepan. Add the teff, cinnamon, cardamom and salt. Stir until mixed. Pour out evenly onto the parchment. Allow to cool, then transfer to a small bowl.

For the syrup, place the tea bags and lavender in a small saucepan with 1 cup (250 mL) of water. Bring to a boil, turn off the heat and let steep for 10 minutes. Strain the liquid, removing the lavender buds and tea bags. Return the liquid to the saucepan and stir in the honey. Bring to a simmer and cook until the liquid has reduced by half and has thickened to a syrupy consistency. Remove from the heat.

Stir the teff to separate it into smaller pieces. Roll tablespoon-sized balls of vanilla ice cream in the mixture until fully coated. Place on a freezer-friendly plate or tray and freeze, uncovered, for at least 15 minutes.

Preheat a barbecue to medium heat, approximately 400°F (200°C).

Continued

ICE CREAM BALLS

1 Tbsp (15 mL) unsalted butter

3 Tbsp (45 mL) lightly packed brown sugar

3 Tbsp (45 mL) teff grains

pinch cinnamon

pinch ground cardamom

pinch salt

½ cup (125 mL) vanilla ice cream

SYRUP

3 chamomile tea bags

¼ tsp (1 mL) food-grade lavender buds

¼ cup (60 mL) liquid honey

PEACHES

3 firm to ripe peaches, halved and pitted

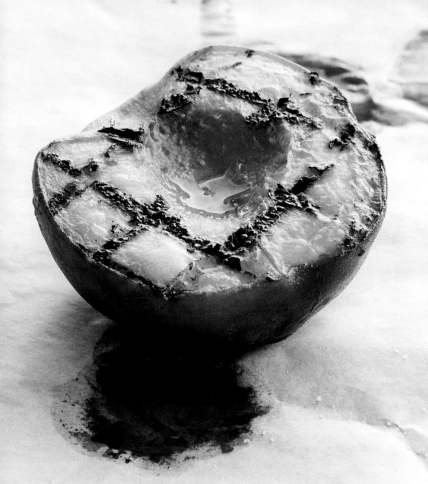

Once the grill is hot, lightly oil it and place the peach halves on it flat side down for 3 minutes. Turn the peaches over and grill the other side for 3 minutes, or until the peaches are warm and tender-firm.

Assemble the dessert by placing a peach half on each plate. Drizzle each with about 1 Tbsp (15 mL) of syrup and top with an ice cream ball. Serve immediately.

Eat this the day you make it.

PER SERVING: Energy 150 calories; Protein 2 g; Carbohydrates 30 g; Dietary Fiber 2 g; Fat 3.5 g; Sugar 21 g; Cholesterol 10 mg; Sodium 60 mg

Strawberry Shortcakes with Sweet Chantilly Cream

To enjoy perfectly ripe strawberries while they are in season you need a good recipe. These tender shortcakes with marinated strawberries and sweet cream will have you truly enjoying summer.

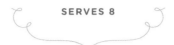

SERVES 8

For the strawberries, place them in a medium bowl with the honey and Grand Marnier, coating them evenly, and set aside.

For the cream, beat the cream and sugar in a stand mixer (or with a handheld mixer in a medium bowl) until stiff peaks form. Cover with plastic wrap and refrigerate until needed.

Line a large baking sheet with parchment paper. Sprinkle the parchment lightly with tapioca starch. Preheat the oven to 400°F (200°C).

For the shortcakes, whisk the tapioca starch, rice and sorghum flours, sugar, baking powder, xanthan gum and salt in a large bowl. Cut in the cold butter with a pastry cutter or pinch it with your fingers until the butter pieces are the size of coarse crumbs.

Pour in the buttermilk and vanilla. Gently stir the mixture with a spatula until the dough comes together. Turn the dough out onto the prepared baking sheet and gently work it with your hands until it's smooth but you can still see pieces of butter. With floured hands, pat the dough into a square 1 inch (2.5 cm) thick. If the dough is too wet, dust it with a small amount of tapioca starch before forming it into a square.

Cut the dough into eight evenly sized shortcakes with a floured pastry cutter or knife. Place them at least 1 ½ inches (4 cm) apart on the baking sheet. Whisk together the egg white and sugar and brush the tops of each biscuit. Sprinkle with almonds. Bake for 15 to 17 minutes, until the shortcakes are golden. Remove from the oven to cool.

To assemble, slice the shortcakes in half and place one half of each on a plate. Divide the strawberries evenly among the shortcake bottoms. Top with a scoop of cream. Replace the tops and serve immediately. Eat these the day you make them.

PER SERVING: Energy 350 calories; Protein 3 g; Carbohydrates 37 g; Dietary Fiber 1 g; Fat 13 g; Sugar 20 g; Cholesterol 25 mg; Sodium 160 mg

STRAWBERRIES

1 lb (450 g) ripe strawberries, hulled and quartered

2 Tbsp (30 mL) liquid honey

1 Tbsp (15 mL) Grand Marnier liqueur

CHANTILLY CREAM

1 cup (250 mL) cold whipping cream

3 Tbsp (45 mL) organic cane sugar or 1 Tbsp (15 mL) liquid honey

SHORTCAKES

⅔ cup (150 mL) tapioca starch, plus extra for dusting

⅔ cup (150 mL) white rice flour

½ cup (125 mL) sorghum flour

⅓ cup (75 mL) organic cane sugar

2 Tbsp (30 mL) baking powder

1 tsp (5 mL) xanthan gum

½ tsp (2 mL) salt

⅓ cup (75 mL) unsalted butter, large cubes, cold

1 cup (250 mL) cold buttermilk (or cold milk-vinegar substitute)

2 tsp (10 mL) pure vanilla extract

1 large egg white

3 Tbsp (45 mL) organic cane sugar

3 Tbsp (45 mL) sliced or slivered almonds

Thai Coconut Dark Chocolate Bark with Lime Zest

Don't feel guilty about eating chocolate! A good-quality dark chocolate can help dilate your arteries and provide a dose of disease-fighting antioxidants. Thai flavors of coconut, chile pepper and lime complement the dark chocolate. Toss in some quinoa crispies and chia seeds and you've added a bit more nutrition too!

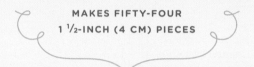

**MAKES FIFTY-FOUR
1 ¹/₂-INCH (4 CM) PIECES**

⅓ cup (75 mL) coarsely chopped unsalted cashews, peanuts or macadamia nuts

1 cup (250 mL) quality semisweet chocolate chips

¼ cup (60 mL) quinoa crispies or quinoa or millet puffs

2 Tbsp (30 mL) unsweetened shredded coconut

1 Tbsp (15 mL) chia seeds

pinch ground cayenne pepper (optional)

1 tsp (5 mL) dried lime zest

Lightly spray with cooking oil or grease a 9-inch (2.5 L) baking pan. Line the bottom with parchment paper and lightly grease the parchment. Preheat the oven to 350°F (180°C).

Place the nuts on a small baking sheet (you can line it with parchment if desired). Bake for 5 to 7 minutes, or until toasted and fragrant. Remove from the oven and set aside on the baking sheet.

Stir the chocolate in a double boiler until melted. Remove from the heat and stir in the quinoa crispies, coconut, chia and cayenne (if using). Pour the mixture into the prepared baking pan and spread it evenly across the bottom. Sprinkle the nuts overtop and gently press them into the chocolate. Sprinkle with the lime zest and let cool in the refrigerator until firm. Break into pieces before serving.

PER SERVING: Energy 20 calories; Protein 0 g; Carbohydrates 2 g; Dietary Fiber 0 g; Fat 1.5 g; Sugar 2 g; Cholesterol 0 mg; Sodium 0 mg

STORAGE

Room Temperature: airtight container, 1 week

Refrigerator: airtight container, 1 week

Candied Ginger, Orange and Pistachio Bark

Dark chocolate combined with ginger, orange and pistachio flavors is divine.
One small piece hits the spot for dessert and provides another nutritious
dose of quinoa or millet and chia.

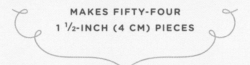

MAKES FIFTY-FOUR
1 ½-INCH (4 CM) PIECES

Lightly grease a 9-inch (2.5 L) square baking pan. Line the bottom with parchment paper and lightly grease the parchment. Preheat the oven to 350°F (180°C).

Place the nuts on a small baking sheet (you can line it with parchment if desired). Bake for 5 to 7 minutes or until toasted and fragrant. Remove from the oven and set aside on the baking sheet.

Melt the chocolate in a double boiler, stirring constantly. Remove from the heat and stir in the quinoa crispies, chia and cardamom. Pour the mixture into the prepared baking pan and spread it evenly across the bottom. Sprinkle the nuts and candied ginger overtop and gently press them into the chocolate. Sprinkle with orange zest and cool in the refrigerator until firm. Break into pieces measuring about 1 ½ inches (4 cm) before serving.

⅓ cup (75 mL) pistachios, coarsely chopped

1 cup (250 mL) quality semisweet chocolate chips

⅓ cup (75 mL) quinoa crispies or quinoa or millet puffs

1 Tbsp (15 mL) chia seeds

pinch ground cardamom

1 Tbsp (15 mL) finely chopped candied ginger

¼ tsp (1 mL) dried orange zest

PER SERVING: Energy 70 calories; Protein 1 g; Carbohydrates 9 g; Dietary Fiber 1 g; Fat 4 g; Sugar 6 g; Cholesterol 0 mg; Sodium 15 mg

STORAGE
Room Temperature: airtight container, 1 week
Refrigerator: airtight container, 1 week

Cherry Almond Truffles

Why wait for a special occasion? These healthy truffles made with oats, quinoa or amaranth, chia, almonds, cherries and dates are good anytime. They're a perfect blend of natural ingredients that can satisfy your cravings for treats. Avoid high-calorie, nutrition-void snacks and make these instead.

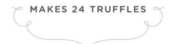

MAKES 24 TRUFFLES

1 cup (250 mL) oat, quinoa or amaranth flakes

1 cup (250 mL) dried sweet cherries

²/₃ cup (150 mL) whole raw almonds

½ cup (125 mL) Medjool dates, pitted

¼ cup (60 mL) cool water

2 Tbsp (30 mL) chia seeds

½ tsp (2 mL) pure vanilla extract

¼ tsp (1 mL) cinnamon

cocoa powder, almond flakes, almond flour or finely shredded unsweetened coconut for rolling

Place the oat flakes, cherries, almonds, dates, water, chia, vanilla and cinnamon in a food processor and pulse until the cherries and dates are pureed but the almonds are still in small pieces.

Using 2 tsp (10 mL) of mixture at a time, form the truffle mixture into balls. Roll in cocoa powder, almond flakes, almond flour or finely shredded unsweetened coconut.

PER SERVING: Energy 70 calories; Protein 2 g; Carbohydrates 11 g; Dietary Fiber 3 g; Fat 2.5 g; Sugar 6 g; Cholesterol 0 mg; Sodium 0 mg

STORAGE

Room Temperature: **airtight container with lid slightly opened, 1 week**

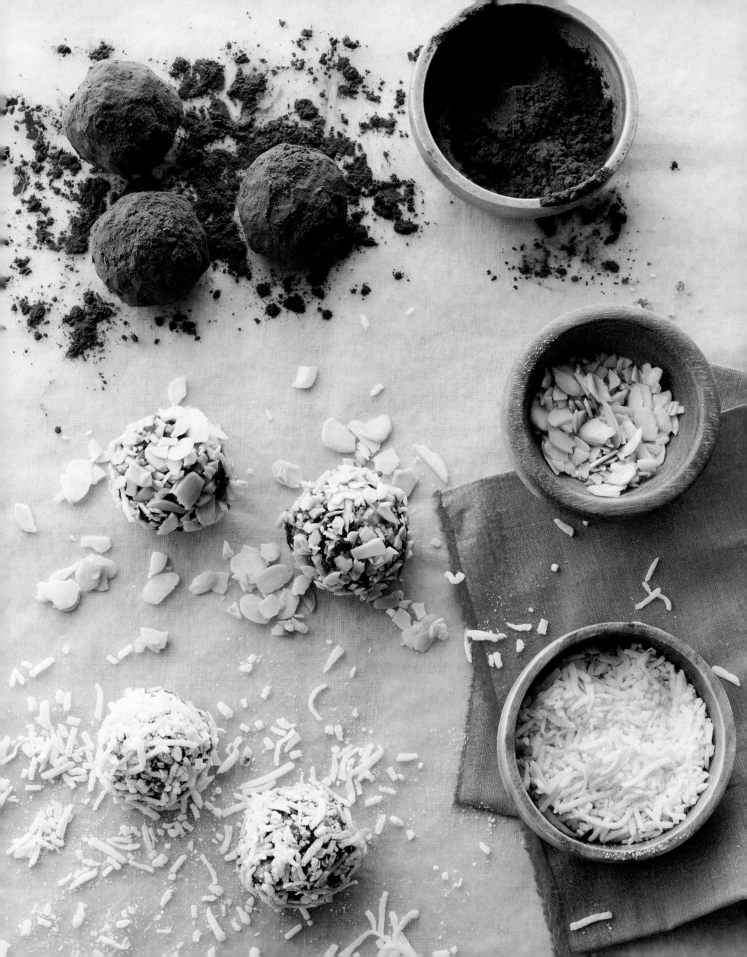

Graham Peanut Butter Chocolate Bites

These no-bake chocolate morsels are made from crumbs of our Graham-Style Wafers recipe (page 46), made with gluten-free ancient grains and peanut butter. The taste is reminiscent of chocolate peanut butter cups and makes a great addition to any tray of after-dinner dessert finger foods.

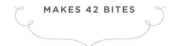

MAKES 42 BITES

¾ cup (175 mL) powdered (icing) sugar

½ cup (125 mL) peanut butter (smooth or chunky) or any other nut butter

3 Tbsp (45 mL) unsalted butter, softened

1 ¼ cups (310 mL) finely crushed Graham-Style Wafers (page 46)

⅔ cup (150 mL) semisweet chocolate chips

Lightly spray with cooking oil or grease a large baking sheet and line with parchment paper.

Beat the sugar, peanut butter and butter together in a medium bowl. Add 1 cup (250 mL) of the crushed Graham-Style Wafers and mix well. Using a teaspoon, scoop up the mixture and roll it into teaspoon-sized (5 mL) balls. Place the remaining ¼ cup (60 mL) of crumbs in a small bowl. Roll each ball in the crumbs and gently flatten each side of the ball to form a cube. Place each cube on the prepared baking sheet and then place in the refrigerator or freezer for 1 hour.

Melt the chocolate chips in a double boiler. Gently dip half of each cube into the melted chocolate. Return to the baking sheet and place in the refrigerator for another hour. Serve cold.

PER SERVING: Energy 60 calories; Protein 1 g; Carbohydrates 6 g; Dietary Fiber 2 g; Fat 3 g; Sugar 4 g; Cholesterol 5 mg; Sodium 15 mg

STORAGE

Room Temperature: **airtight container, 1 week**

Refrigerator: **airtight container, 1 week**

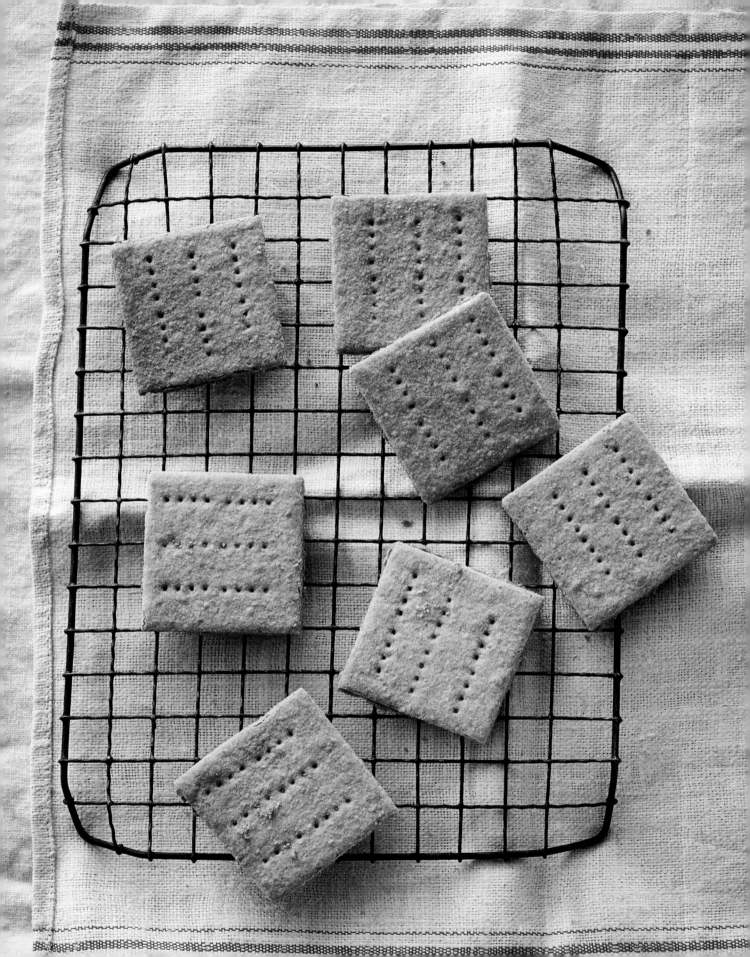

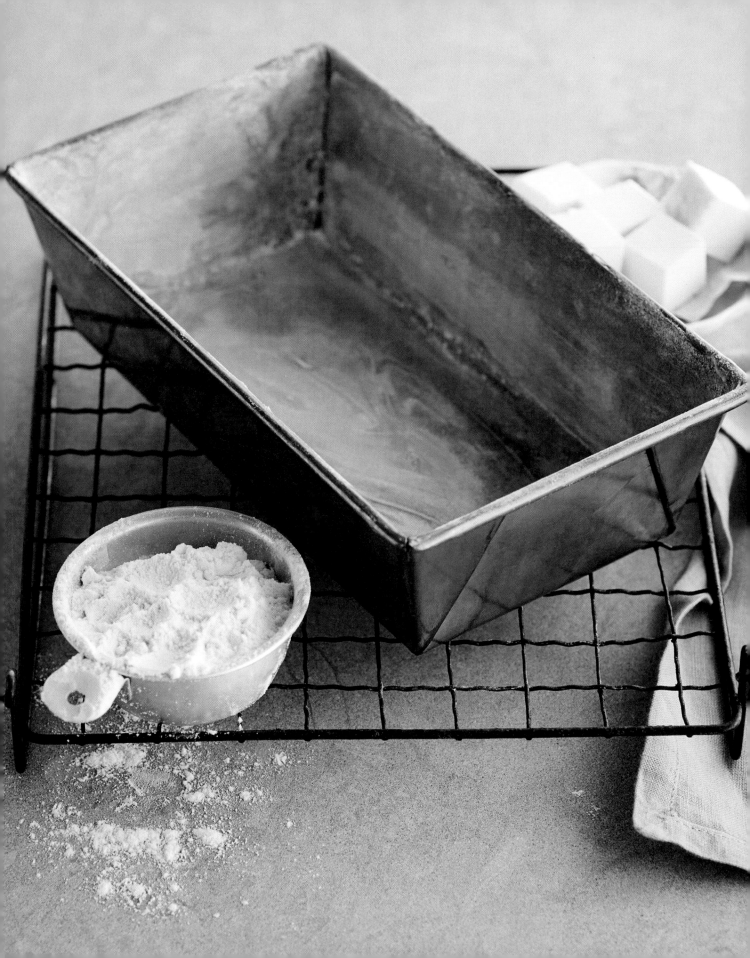

Savory Breads and Buns

Enriched White Bread   162

French Bread   164

Tender Egg Bread (Challah)   166

Dill Cilantro Buttermilk Bread with Mint   167

Ancient Grain Bread   169

Molasses Ancient Grain Loaf   170

Chipotle Cheddar Quick Bread   172

Basil Pesto and Pine Nut Loaf   173

Roasted Red Pepper Loaf   175

Ancient Grain Tortilla Wraps   176

Multigrain Buns   178

White Dinner Buns   180

Homemade Soft Pretzels   182

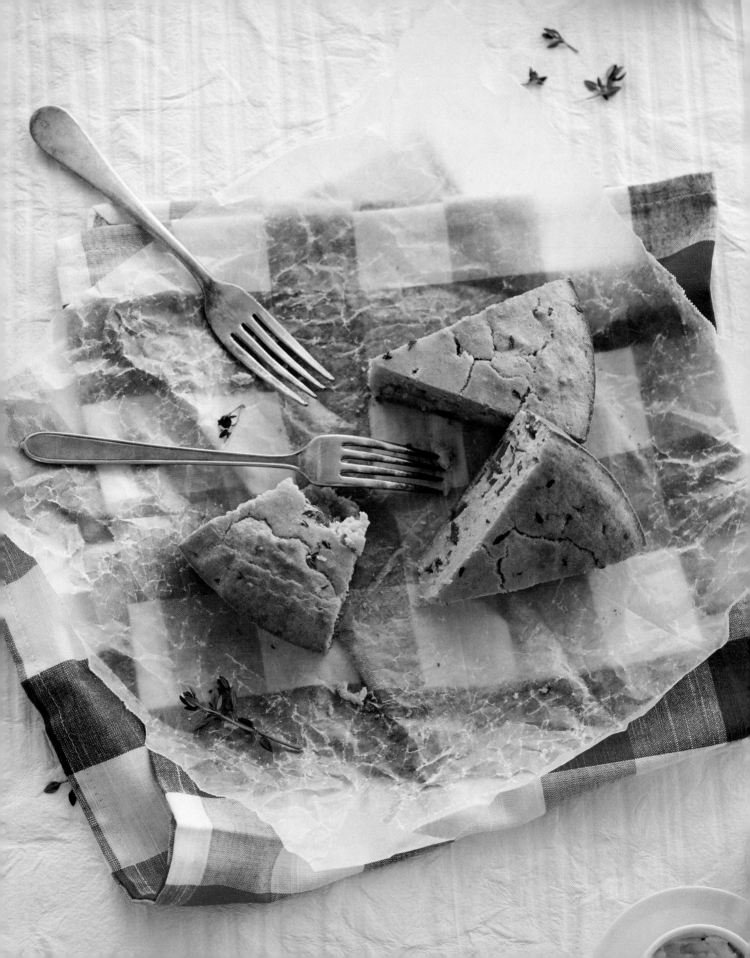

Bread is a staple for many of us, and has been for many generations. For some people, it seems hard to live without. Comforting and familiar, breads can enhance your whole meal. You don't have to miss out on breads just because you're eating gluten-free. They do not have to be made with wheat or gluten flours! And gluten-free breads do not have to be made exclusively from combinations of ingredients like rice flours, starches, gums and pectin. Delicious, healthy and fluffy soft bread is possible using a range of nutritious gluten-free ingredients, even better than any bread you can buy at a bakery or grocery store. You can have breads that are full of fiber and whole grains and loaded with natural vitamins and minerals.

Served warm or cold, gluten-free breads can be comforting and wholesome and make quick meals on their own — such as sandwiches — or be sides for soups, casseroles or salads.

Remember when making yeast breads that they need to rise in a warm place. Cover them well and protect them from drafts, even if it means placing them inside a cupboard!

The lack of preservatives in home-baked breads gives them a short shelf-life. Freezing is a terrific option, especially for maintaining the freshness of bread and buns. After baking, cool the goods completely in the open air for at least 4 hours before freezing in resealable plastic bags. Loaves of bread (unless you are going to use an entire loaf in one day) are best cooled, sliced and frozen. Some people prefer to place parchment between each slice for easy removal.

Baked and frozen bread and buns are best thawed at room temperature for 20 to 30 minutes, then reheated for 10 to 15 minutes at 325°F (160°C). If you want to bake the dough from a frozen state, bake it at 400°F (200°C) for 5 to 9 minutes. Wrap soft, crusted breads such as Molasses Ancient Grain Loaf (page 170) in aluminum foil prior to baking to prevent them from getting too crusty. Overall, reheating the bread or buns in the oven makes for a fresher loaf.

For a fabulous sandwich loaf that is as good as any regular bread, try the Enriched White Bread (page 162); for awesome dinner buns, try the White Dinner Buns (page 180). If you're the whole wheat type, try the Multigrain Buns (page 178) or the moist and light Ancient Grain Bread (page 169). For a hit of flavor, try the Chipotle Cheddar Quick Bread (page 172) or Roasted Red Pepper Loaf (page 175). Handheld delights include our Homemade Soft Pretzels (page 182) and Ancient Grain Tortilla Wraps (page 176), which are better than any store-bought soft tortillas!

Enriched White Bread

White bread itself is not very nutritious, but we have enriched this recipe with sorghum, chia and psyllium so you can enjoy an occasional slice or two of white bread that is gluten-free. Use this for your favorite sandwiches or toast for breakfast.

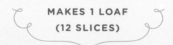

**MAKES 1 LOAF
(12 SLICES)**

1 cup (250 mL) sorghum flour

³/₄ cup (175 mL) tapioca starch

³/₄ cup (175 mL) potato starch

¹/₂ cup (125 mL) white rice flour

¹/₄ cup (60 mL) ground chia seeds

3 Tbsp (45 mL) psyllium husks

2 tsp (10 mL) xanthan gum

2 Tbsp (30 mL) organic cane sugar

1 Tbsp (15 mL) quick-rising yeast

1 ¹/₂ tsp (7 mL) salt

¹/₂ tsp (2 mL) cream of tartar

1 ¹/₂ cups (375 mL) warm 1% milk or milk substitute at 120–125°F (50–52°C)

2 large eggs

2 Tbsp (30 mL) grapeseed or organic light-tasting oil

1 tsp (5 mL) apple cider vinegar

Lightly grease a 9- × 5-inch (2 L) loaf pan. Line the sides and bottom with one piece of parchment paper and lightly grease the parchment.

Combine the sorghum flour, tapioca starch, potato starch, rice flour, chia, psyllium, xanthan gum, sugar, yeast, salt and cream of tartar in the bowl of a stand mixer using the paddle attachment or a whisk, or in a large bowl (if using a handheld mixer). Whisk until all the ingredients are mixed together. Pour in the warm milk and use the paddle attachment to stir the ingredients together on low speed. Add the eggs, oil and apple cider vinegar. Mix on a medium setting for 4 to 5 minutes. The dough should be sticky and thick.

Turn the dough into the loaf pan using an oiled spatula. Level the dough, then slightly mound into the shape of a loaf top. Cover with a damp cloth and place in a warm, draft-free spot to rise until doubled in size, about 50 minutes.

Preheat the oven to 375°F (190°C).

Bake the bread for 55 to 65 minutes, or until an instant read thermometer reads 205°F (96°C). Cover the loaf with aluminum foil during baking when the bread reaches the perfect golden color. Start checking around 25 minutes into the baking time. Remove from the oven, discard the foil and carefully tip the bread out of the pan onto a cooling rack. Let it rest, mounded side up, for 10 minutes before using. Freeze the bread after it has cooled completely (at least 4 hours).

PER SERVING: Energy 220 calories; Protein 5 g; Carbohydrates 40 g; Dietary Fiber 6 g; Fat 5 g; Sugar 4 g; Cholesterol 35 mg; Sodium 220 mg

STORAGE

Room Temperature: **airtight container or bag, 2 days**

Refrigerator: **airtight container or bag, 4 days**

Freezer: **airtight freezer bag or container, 1 month**

Baked Seasoned Croutons

Enhance meals with gluten-free croutons from your own kitchen. They are a cost-effective, delicious alternative to the pre-packaged ones. And they're quick to make. Adjust the flavor as you like. The herbs are optional. White or French bread croutons are the most versatile.

4 cups (1 L) ½-inch (1.5 cm) bread cubes, any type of bread

3 Tbsp (45 mL) butter or olive oil

1 ½ tsp (7 mL) chopped fresh thyme (optional)

½ tsp (2 mL) chopped fresh rosemary (optional)

¼ tsp (1 mL) finely chopped garlic

¼ tsp (1 mL) salt (optional)

Preheat the oven to 325°F (160°C). Set a large, unlined rimmed baking sheet aside.

Place the bread cubes in a large bowl and set aside. In a small saucepan on the stovetop, heat the butter or oil until melted or very warm. Remove from the heat and stir in the herbs (if using), garlic and salt (if using). Toss the butter/oil mixture into the bread cubes, mixing until evenly distributed. Spread the cubes in an even layer (without any touching) on the rimmed baking sheet and bake for 10 minutes. Turn once and bake for another 10 minutes, until dry and golden. Cool completely.

STORAGE

Room Temperature: airtight container or bag, 2 weeks

Freezer: airtight freezer bag or container, 1 month

Bread Crumbs or Cubes

Don't waste time searching for gluten-free bread crumbs and cubes in stores. Have them ready as you need them and prevent the needless waste of crusts and unused bread by making your own. Collect, chop and dry bread cubes on an ongoing basis. Grind them into crumbs when you have several dried cubes or as you need them.

Any amount of French or white bread, cut into approximately 1-inch (2.5 cm) pieces

Dry the cubes of bread over several hours in a single layer on a baking sheet at room temperature or in the oven at 275°F (135°C) for 10 to 15 minutes, then cool completely. To make crumbs, pulse the dried bread cubes in a food processor or blender until the desired crumb size is reached. Use as desired.

French Bread

This French bread can be used for many things, including garlic bread or sandwiches, or as an addition to a cheese platter. Use it to complement a continental breakfast or anywhere you'd serve French bread. Freeze the baked loaves after they have cooled completely, at least 4 hours.

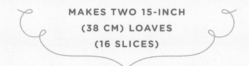

MAKES TWO 15-INCH (38 CM) LOAVES (16 SLICES)

1 cup (250 mL) sorghum flour

1 cup (250 mL) tapioca starch, plus extra for forming dough

½ cup (125 mL) white rice flour

½ cup (125 mL) potato starch

¼ cup (60 mL) ground chia seeds

3 Tbsp (45 mL) psyllium husks

2 tsp (10 mL) xanthan gum

2 Tbsp (30 mL) organic cane sugar

1 Tbsp (15 mL) quick-rising yeast

1 ½ tsp (7 mL) salt

½ tsp (2 mL) cream of tartar

1 ¼ cups (310 mL) warm 1% milk or milk substitute at 120–125°F (50–52°C)

2 large eggs

2 Tbsp (30 mL) grapeseed or organic light-tasting oil

Line a large baking sheet with parchment paper.

Combine the sorghum flour, tapioca starch, rice flour, potato starch, chia, psyllium, xanthan gum, sugar, yeast, salt and cream of tartar in the bowl of a stand mixer, using a paddle attachment or a whisk, or a large bowl (if using a handheld mixer). Whisk until all the ingredients are mixed together. Pour in the warm milk and use the paddle attachment (or a handheld mixer) to stir the ingredients together on low speed. Add the eggs and oil. Mix on a medium setting for 4 to 5 minutes. The dough should be sticky but not gooey.

Flour your hands. Divide the dough in half and roll each half into a ball. Roll one piece on a lightly floured surface until it is 15 inches (38 cm) long. Slice three diagonal shallow lines in the top and set it on the parchment. Repeat with the second piece. Cover them and place them in a warm, draft-free spot to rise until doubled in size, about 50 minutes.

Preheat the oven to 375°F (190°C).

Bake the loaves for 40 minutes, or until an instant read thermometer reads 205°F (96°C). Cover the loaves with aluminum foil during baking when the bread reaches the perfect golden color. Start checking around 25 minutes into the baking time. Remove from the oven, discard the foil and let the loaves rest on the baking sheet for 10 minutes before using.

PER SERVING: Energy 110 calories; Protein 2 g; Carbohydrates 19 g; Dietary Fiber 2 g; Fat 2 g; Sugar 2 g; Cholesterol 15 mg; Sodium 160 mg

STORAGE

Room Temperature: airtight container or bag, 2 days

Refrigerator: airtight container or bag, 4 days

Freezer: airtight freezer bag or container, 1 month

Freezer Garlic Bread

Make these fabulous pieces of garlic bread ahead of time, freeze them and have individual pieces ready to go in a snap. Just bake, serve and enjoy. Add a sprinkle of cheese, if desired.

1 loaf of French Bread, cooled completely at room temperature (4 hours minimum)

¼ cup (60 mL) salted butter

1 ½ tsp (7 mL) finely chopped garlic

¼ tsp (1 mL) salt

pinch ground black pepper

Line a baking sheet or tray that will fit in the freezer with parchment paper.

Slice the loaf into 10 pieces. Mix together the butter, garlic, salt and pepper. Spread some of this butter mixture on one side of each piece of bread. Place the bread, butter side up, on the baking sheet and freeze completely (3 hours). Remove from the freezer and place in a resealable plastic bag. Return to the freezer for up to 3 weeks. When ready to use, bake the pieces in a preheated oven at 425°F (220°C) for 8 to 10 minutes, until hot and the edges are golden. Serve immediately.

Pizza Bread

Delicious cheesy, tomato pizza is an all-time flavor favorite. Make this bread and serve it as an appetizer or part of a meal.

Preheat the oven to 400°F (200°C).

Cut a loaf of French bread in half lengthwise. Spread with your choice of pizza sauce, desired toppings and shredded mozzarella cheese.

Bake for 10 to 20 minutes (depending on the amount of toppings). If you are using several veggies, you may want to sauté them first to reduce the baking time. Cut the pizza bread into the desired portions and serve immediately.

Crostini

Create your own bite-sized, toasted crostini! Ready for endless topping combinations and great for appetizers such as bruschetta, or with tapenade and cheeses. Enjoy them in soups or with your favorite dips.

Preheat the oven to 325°F (160°C).

Slice your bread (any bread) into ½-inch (1 cm) thick slices (quarter slices of full-sized, store-bought loaves). Place the slices in a single layer on a baking sheet. If desired, brush them lightly with olive oil and rub with a halved piece of garlic for enhanced flavor before baking. Bake for 5 to 10 minutes, until dry and slightly golden. Remove from the oven and use as desired.

STORAGE
Room Temperature: airtight container or bag, 1 week
Freezer: airtight freezer bag or container, 1 month

Tender Egg Bread (Challah)

Slightly sweet and tender, this delicate, gluten-free bread is made in a Bundt pan. It is inspired by challah bread and is a lovely golden color.

**MAKES 1 LOAF
(8 SERVINGS)**

2 tsp (10 mL) sesame seeds

½ cup (125 mL) oat flour

½ cup (125 mL) tapioca starch

½ cup (125 mL) white rice flour

⅓ cup (75 mL) cornstarch

3 Tbsp (45 mL) organic cane sugar

1 Tbsp (15 mL) quick-rising yeast

1 ½ Tbsp (7 mL) psyllium husks

1 tsp (5 mL) xanthan gum

¼ tsp (1 mL) salt

½ cup (125 mL) warm 1% milk or milk substitute at 120–125°F (50–52°C)

2 large eggs

⅓ cup (75 mL) olive oil

Lightly grease a 9-inch (3 L) Bundt pan and sprinkle it with the sesame seeds.

Whisk together the oat flour, tapioca starch, rice flour, cornstarch, sugar, yeast, psyllium, xanthan gum and salt in a stand mixer bowl or large bowl. Add the warm milk, mixing it into the flours until evenly distributed. Set aside. Whisk together the eggs and oil in a medium bowl. Add to the ingredients in the mixer or bowl and mix for 4 minutes on a medium setting.

Pour the dough into the pan, using a spatula to spread it evenly. Cover with a slightly damp kitchen towel and let it rise in a warm, draft-free place until doubled in size, 1 hour.

Preheat the oven to 350°F (180°C).

Bake the bread for 20 minutes. Remove from the oven, carefully turn out the bread and place it flat side down on a baking sheet. Bake for an additional 10 minutes, or until a thermometer inserted in the center reads 205°F (96°C). Allow to cool for 10 minutes, then cover with a dry kitchen towel to keep warm until ready to serve.

PER SERVING: Energy 250 calories; Protein 4 g; Carbohydrates 32 g; Dietary Fiber 4 g; Fat 10 g; Sugar 6 g; Cholesterol 45 mg; Sodium 100 mg

BAKING TIP
Make French toast with any of the leftover breads in this chapter, including Tender Egg Bread.

STORAGE
Room Temperature: airtight container or bag, 1 day
Refrigerator: airtight container or bag, 1 day

Dill Cilantro Buttermilk Bread with Mint

Enriched with quinoa, oat and sorghum flours, this moist and fluffy white loaf is made with buttermilk, cream cheese and fresh herbs. This is perfect alongside stew, chili or any soup.

**MAKES 2 LOAVES
(12 SLICES EACH)**

Lightly grease or spray with cooking oil two 9- × 5-inch (2 L) loaf pans. Line the pans with parchment paper. Preheat the oven to 350°F (180°C).

Whisk together the quinoa, oat and sorghum flours, tapioca starch, baking powder and salt in a medium bowl. Cut in the butter and cream cheese until the mixture resembles large crumbs. Set aside.

In a separate medium bowl, whisk together the buttermilk, eggs, dill, cilantro and mint. Gently add all the buttermilk mixture to the flour mixture and fold it in until the flour is just moist. Divide the dough between each prepared loaf pan.

Bake for 35 to 40 minutes, until a toothpick inserted into the center comes out clean. Let the loaves cool slightly in the pans before moving them to a wire rack to completely cool. Slice while still warm, or wait until they have cooled completely, if you prefer.

PER SERVING: Energy 160 calories; Protein 4 g; Carbohydrates 18 g; Dietary Fiber 2 g; Fat 8 g; Sugar 1 g; Cholesterol 65 mg; Sodium 90 mg

1 cup (250 mL) quinoa flour

½ cup (125 mL) oat flour

½ cup (125 mL) sorghum flour

1 cup (250 mL) tapioca starch

1 ½ Tbsp (22 mL) baking powder

¼ tsp (1 mL) salt

⅓ cup (75 mL) cold, unsalted butter

⅓ cup (75 mL) cold cream cheese

1 cup (250 mL) buttermilk (or milk-vinegar substitute)

4 large eggs

1 Tbsp (15 mL) chopped fresh dill

1 Tbsp (15 mL) chopped fresh cilantro

1 Tbsp (15 mL) chopped fresh mint

STORAGE
Room Temperature: airtight container or bag, 1 day
Refrigerator: airtight container or bag, 3 days

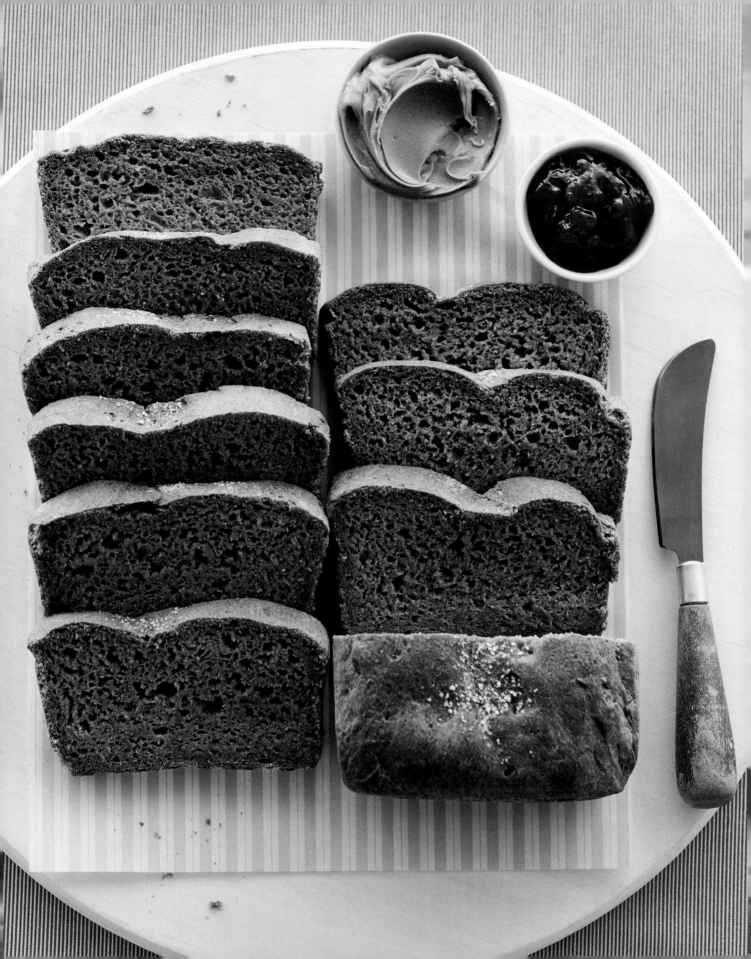

Ancient Grain Bread

Whole wheat bread has met its match! This beautifully brown, moist, light sandwich loaf is made wholesome and gluten-free with teff, buckwheat and chia. Terrific for your favorite sandwiches, it also toasts nicely for breakfast.

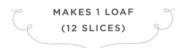

**MAKES 1 LOAF
(12 SLICES)**

Lightly grease a 9- × 5-inch (2 L) loaf pan. Line the sides and bottom with one piece of parchment and lightly grease the parchment.

Combine the teff and buckwheat flours, tapioca and potato starches, chia, psyllium, xanthan gum, sugar, yeast, salt and cream of tartar in the bowl of a stand mixer or large bowl (if using a handheld mixer). Stir all the ingredients together using a paddle attachment or whisk. Pour in the warm milk and use the paddle attachment (or a large spatula) to stir the ingredients together. Add the eggs, oil and apple cider vinegar. Continue to mix on medium speed for 4 to 5 minutes. The dough should be sticky and thick. Turn the dough into the loaf pan using an oiled spatula. Level off the dough, then slightly mound it into the shape of a loaf top. Place it in a warm, draft-free area, covered with a dry towel, until doubled in size, about 50 minutes.

Preheat the oven to 375°F (190°C).

Bake the loaf for 55 to 65 minutes, or until an instant read thermometer inserted in the center reads 205°F (96°C). Cover the loaf with aluminum foil during baking when the bread reaches the perfect golden color and you do not want further browning. Start checking around 25 minutes into the baking time. Remove from the oven, discard the foil and carefully tip the bread out of the pan onto a cooling rack. Let it rest, mounded side up, for 10 minutes before using.

PER SERVING: Energy 190 calories; Protein 5 g; Carbohydrates 33 g; Dietary Fiber 4 g; Fat 5 g; Sugar 4 g; Cholesterol 35 mg; Sodium 180 mg

¾ cup (175 mL) teff flour

⅔ cup (150 mL) light buckwheat flour

¾ cup (175 mL) tapioca starch

¾ cup (175 mL) potato starch

¼ cup (60 mL) ground chia seeds

3 Tbsp (45 mL) psyllium husks

2 tsp (10 mL) xanthan gum

2 Tbsp (30 mL) organic cane sugar

1 Tbsp (15 mL) quick-rising yeast

1 ½ tsp (7 mL) salt

½ tsp (2 mL) cream of tartar

1 ½ cups (375 mL) warm 1% milk or milk substitute at 120–125°F (50–52°C)

2 large eggs

2 Tbsp (30 mL) grapeseed or organic light-tasting oil

1 tsp (5 mL) apple cider vinegar

STORAGE

Room Temperature: airtight container or bag, 3 days

Refrigerator: airtight container or bag, 4 days

Freezer: airtight freezer bag or container, 2 weeks

Molasses Ancient Grain Loaf

The rich, comforting flavor and texture of this loaf brings a new dimension to bread. Buckwheat, sorghum and quinoa flour add complete proteins and whole, ancient grain goodness to this hardy loaf. Eat it in sandwiches, toasted with cream cheese or with cheese and fresh fruit.

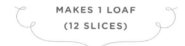

**MAKES 1 LOAF
(12 SLICES)**

¾ cup (175 mL) light
    buckwheat flour

¾ cup (175 mL) sorghum flour

¾ cup (175 mL) quinoa flour

¾ cup (175 mL) sweet rice flour

¼ cup (60 mL) psyllium husks

1 Tbsp (15 mL) xanthan gum

1 Tbsp (15 mL) baking powder

1 ½ tsp (7 mL) salt

¼ tsp (1 mL) baking soda

½ tsp (2 mL) cream of tartar

3 large eggs

2 ¼ cups (560 mL) buttermilk
    (or milk-vinegar substitute)

¾ cup (175 mL) fancy molasses

Lightly grease a 9- × 5-inch (2 L) loaf pan. Line the bottom and sides with one piece of parchment paper and lightly grease the parchment. Preheat the oven to 350°F (180°C).

Whisk together the buckwheat, sorghum, quinoa and sweet rice flours, psyllium, xanthan gum, baking powder, salt, baking soda and cream of tartar in a large bowl until blended. Make a well in the center and set aside.

Lightly whisk the eggs in a medium bowl. Continue to whisk as you add the buttermilk and molasses. Pour the liquid into the well of the dry ingredients. Stir until combined. Scrape the dough into the loaf pan using an oiled spatula. Level off the dough, then slightly mound it into the shape of a loaf top.

Bake for 55 to 60 minutes. Place aluminum foil over the loaf halfway through the baking process to prevent overbrowning. Remove from the oven when an instant read thermometer inserted in the center reads 205°F (96°C). The bread should be dark golden in color. Remove from the oven, discard the foil and carefully tip the loaf out of the pan onto a cooling rack. Let it rest, mounded side up, for 10 minutes before slicing.

PER SERVING: Energy 220 calories; Protein 6 g; Carbohydrates 39 g; Dietary Fiber 8 g; Fat 3 g; Sugar 7 g; Cholesterol 50 mg; Sodium 190 mg

STORAGE
Room Temperature: **airtight container or bag, 3 days**
Refrigerator: **airtight container or bag, 3 days**
Freezer: **airtight freezer bag or container, 2 weeks**

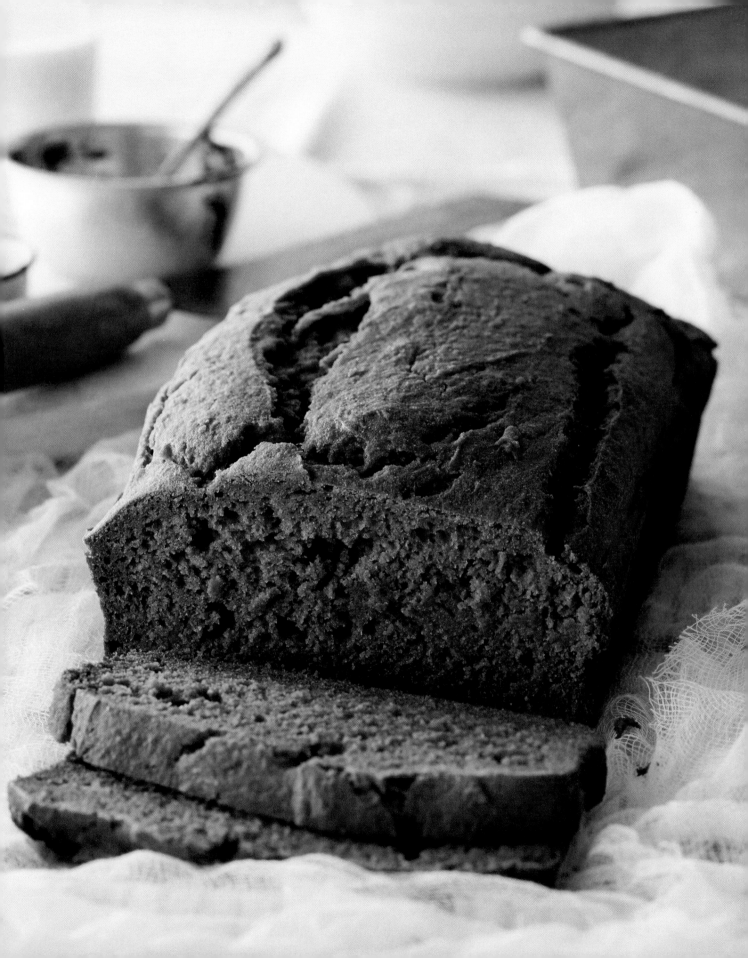

Chipotle Cheddar Quick Bread

*Enjoy a homemade chili, salad, soup or stew with a piece of warm
Chipotle Cheddar Quick Bread made with sorghum and millet ancient grains.*

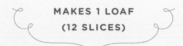

**MAKES 1 LOAF
(12 SLICES)**

1 ¼ cups (310 mL) grated sharp
Cheddar cheese

1 cup (250 mL) sorghum flour

1 cup (250 mL) tapioca starch

½ cup (125 mL) organic cornmeal

¼ cup (60 mL) millet flour

2 tsp (10 mL) xanthan gum

1 Tbsp (15 mL) organic cane sugar

1 ½ tsp (7 mL) baking powder

½ tsp (2 mL) baking soda

¾ tsp (3 mL) ground chipotle
pepper

¾ tsp (3 mL) salt

⅓ cup (75 mL) sliced green
onions

2 large eggs

1 ½ cups (310 mL) buttermilk (or
milk-vinegar substitute)

3 Tbsp (45 mL) grapeseed or
organic light-tasting oil

Lightly grease a 9- × 5-inch (2 L) loaf pan. Line the bottom
and sides with one piece of parchment paper and lightly grease
the parchment or spray with cooking oil. Scatter 2 Tbsp (30 mL)
of the cheese over the bottom of the pan. Preheat the oven to
350°F (180°C).

Whisk together the sorghum flour, tapioca starch, cornmeal,
millet flour, xanthan gum, sugar, baking powder, baking soda,
chipotle pepper and salt in a large bowl until blended. Stir in
1 cup (250 mL) of the cheese and the green onions until
evenly distributed. Make a well in the center and set aside.

Lightly whisk the eggs in a small bowl, then whisk in the
buttermilk and oil. Pour the liquid into the well of the dry
ingredients. Stir until just combined. Pour into the prepared
loaf pan and use an oiled spatula to level off the dough, then
mound it into the shape of a loaf top. Sprinkle with the
remaining 2 Tbsp (30 mL) of cheese.

Bake for 55 to 60 minutes, until an instant read thermometer
inserted in the center reads 205°F (96°C). The bread should
be golden in color. If the top of the bread reaches a deep golden
color prior to being completely baked, cover with aluminum foil
for the remainder of the baking process. Start checking 25 minutes
into the baking time. Remove from the oven, discard the foil and
carefully tip the bread out of the pan onto a cooling rack. Let it
rest, mounded side up, for 10 minutes before slicing.

PER SERVING: Energy 190 calories; Protein 7 g; Carbohydrates 27 g;
Dietary Fiber 2 g; Fat 6 g; Sugar 3 g; Cholesterol 35 mg; Sodium 280 mg

STORAGE

Room Temperature: airtight container or bag, 2 days

Refrigerator: airtight container or bag, 2 days

Freezer: airtight freezer bag or container, 2 weeks

Basil Pesto and Pine Nut Loaf

This fluffy, round loaf, cut into wedges, is perfect alongside a bowl of soup or stew.
It's made with ancient grains — sorghum, oat and millet flours —
and flavored with zesty pesto, pine nuts and freshly chopped basil.

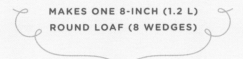

**MAKES ONE 8-INCH (1.2 L)
ROUND LOAF (8 WEDGES)**

Lightly grease or spray with cooking oil an 8-inch (1 L) round cake pan. Line the pan with parchment paper. Preheat the oven to 350°F (180°C).

Whisk together the sorghum, oat and millet flours, tapioca starch, baking powder and salt in a medium bowl. Set aside.

In a separate medium bowl, whisk together the eggs, buttermilk, oil, yogurt, pesto, pine nuts and basil. Add all the buttermilk mixture to the flour mixture and gently fold it in until the flour is just moist. Pour the dough into the prepared baking pan.

Bake for 30 to 35 minutes, until a toothpick inserted into the center comes out clean and the top and edges are slightly golden. Let the loaf cool slightly in the pan before turning it out onto a cutting surface and slicing into wedges. Serve warm.

Best eaten the day you make it.

PER SERVING: Energy 260 calories; Protein 7 g; Carbohydrates 24 g; Dietary Fiber 3 g; Fat 11 g; Sugar 2 g; Cholesterol 50 mg; Sodium 240 mg

¾ cup (175 mL) sorghum flour

¾ cup (175 mL) oat flour

½ cup (125 mL) millet flour

¼ cup (60 mL) tapioca starch

1 Tbsp (15 mL) baking powder

½ tsp (1 mL) salt

2 large eggs

1 cup (250 mL) buttermilk
(or milk-vinegar substitute)

⅓ cup (75 mL) grapeseed oil

¼ cup (60 mL) plain yogurt

2 Tbsp (30 mL) fresh or prepared basil pesto

2 Tbsp (30 mL) pine nuts

2 Tbsp (30 mL) chopped fresh basil leaves

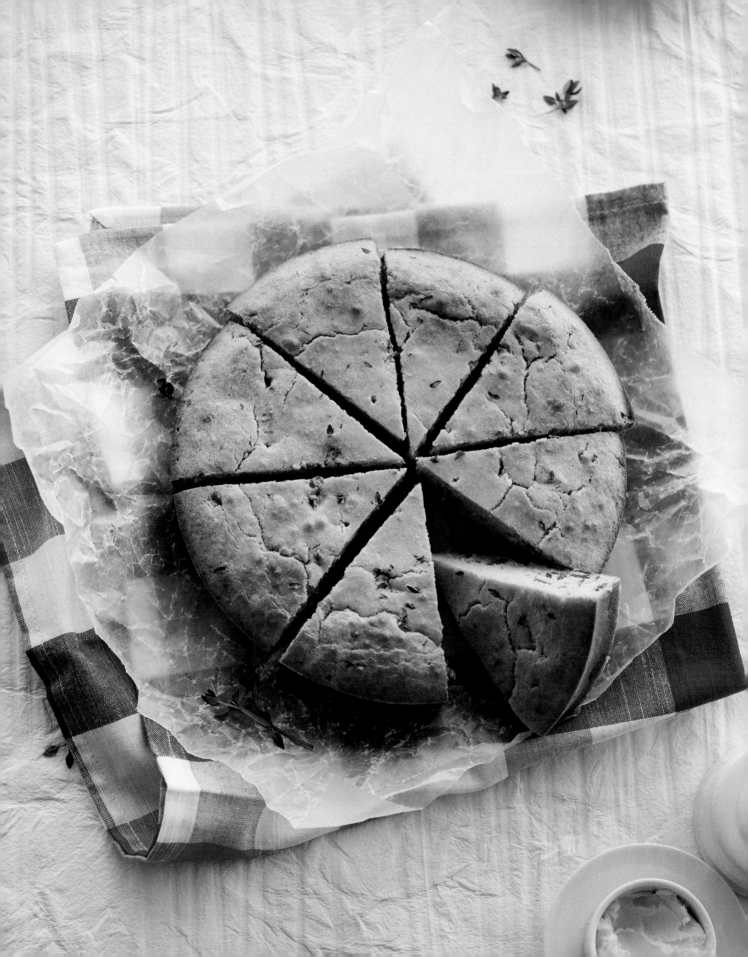

Roasted Red Pepper Loaf

*This is a light and airy bread made of sorghum, oat and millet flours tossed
with generous amounts of chopped roasted red peppers and fresh thyme.*

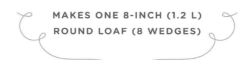

**MAKES ONE 8-INCH (1.2 L)
ROUND LOAF (8 WEDGES)**

Lightly grease or spray with cooking oil an 8-inch (1 L) round
cake pan. Line the pan with parchment paper. Preheat the oven
to 375°F (190°C).

Whisk together the sorghum, millet and oat flours, tapioca
starch, baking powder and salt in a medium bowl. Set aside.

In a separate medium bowl, whisk together the egg yolks,
buttermilk, oil, yogurt, sugar, red peppers and thyme. Add all
the buttermilk mixture to the flour mixture and gently fold it
in until the flour is just moist.

In another bowl, beat the egg whites on high speed until stiff
peaks form. Gently fold them into the dough. Pour the dough
into the prepared baking pan.

Bake for 38 to 40 minutes, until a toothpick inserted into
the center comes out clean. Let the loaf cool slightly in the pan
before turning it out onto a cutting surface and slicing into
wedges. Serve warm.

PER SERVING: Energy 230 calories; Protein 6 g; Carbohydrates 30 g;
Dietary Fiber 2 g; Fat 9 g; Sugar 5 g; Cholesterol 50 mg; Sodium 210 mg

½ cup (125 mL) sorghum flour

½ cup (125 mL) millet flour

½ cup (125 mL) oat flour

½ cup (125 mL) tapioca starch

2 tsp (10 mL) baking powder

¼ tsp (1 mL) salt

2 large eggs, separated

1 cup (250 mL) buttermilk
(or milk-vinegar substitute)

¼ cup (60 mL) grapeseed oil

¼ cup (60 mL) plain yogurt

2 Tbsp (30 mL) organic
cane sugar

¾ cup (175 mL) chopped roasted
red peppers

2 Tbsp (30 mL) chopped fresh
thyme

Ancient Grain Tortilla Wraps

These tender, soft and nutritious tortillas are made with sorghum and teff ancient grains. Their light flavor makes them perfect for quesadillas, burritos and wraps. Best eaten fresh, but may be frozen as pre-made burritos and gently reheated.

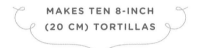

MAKES TEN 8-INCH (20 CM) TORTILLAS

1 cup (250 mL) tapioca starch, with extra for dusting

²/₃ cup (150 mL) sorghum flour

2 Tbsp (30 mL) teff flour

4 tsp (20 mL) psyllium husks

½ tsp (2 mL) salt

2 Tbsp (30 mL) unsalted butter, softened

²/₃ cup + 2 Tbsp (180 mL) room-temperature water

Draw an 8-inch (20 cm) circle onto a large resealable plastic bag using a permanent marker and cut the sides but leave the bottom seam intact. You're going to roll the dough inside this.

Whisk the tapioca starch, sorghum and teff flours, psyllium and salt together in a medium bowl until blended. Work in the butter with your hands until it's evenly distributed. Add the ²/₃ cup (150 mL) water, working it in until you have a dough. Form the dough into a ball, wrap tightly in plastic wrap and let sit for 15 minutes. Add the remaining 2 Tbsp (30 mL) of water and work it into the dough. The dough should not stick to your hands or crack when pressed. (If the dough seems too sticky, add a bit more tapioca starch. If it cracks, add a bit more water.)

Divide the dough into 10 equal pieces, roll them into balls and cover them with a damp towel to prevent drying. Lightly dust the inside of the plastic bag circle with tapioca starch and place a piece of dough in the center. Dust the top of the dough and place the top of the plastic bag circle over the dough. Roll it into an 8-inch (20 cm) circle about ⅛ inch (0.3 cm) thick, dusting each side of the tortilla halfway through rolling.

Warm a 10-inch (25 cm) cast iron skillet or sauté pan over medium heat. Place the tortilla in the warm, dry pan and cook for 20 seconds before flipping to the other side. Place the tortilla on a plate and cover with a clean, slightly damp towel. Repeat with the remaining dough. Use the tortillas as desired.

Best eaten the day you make them.

PER SERVING: Energy 110 calories; Protein 1 g; Carbohydrates 22 g; Dietary Fiber 3 g; Fat 3 g; Sugar 0 g; Cholesterol 5 mg; Sodium 120 mg

STORAGE

Freezer: **airtight freezer bag, 2 weeks**

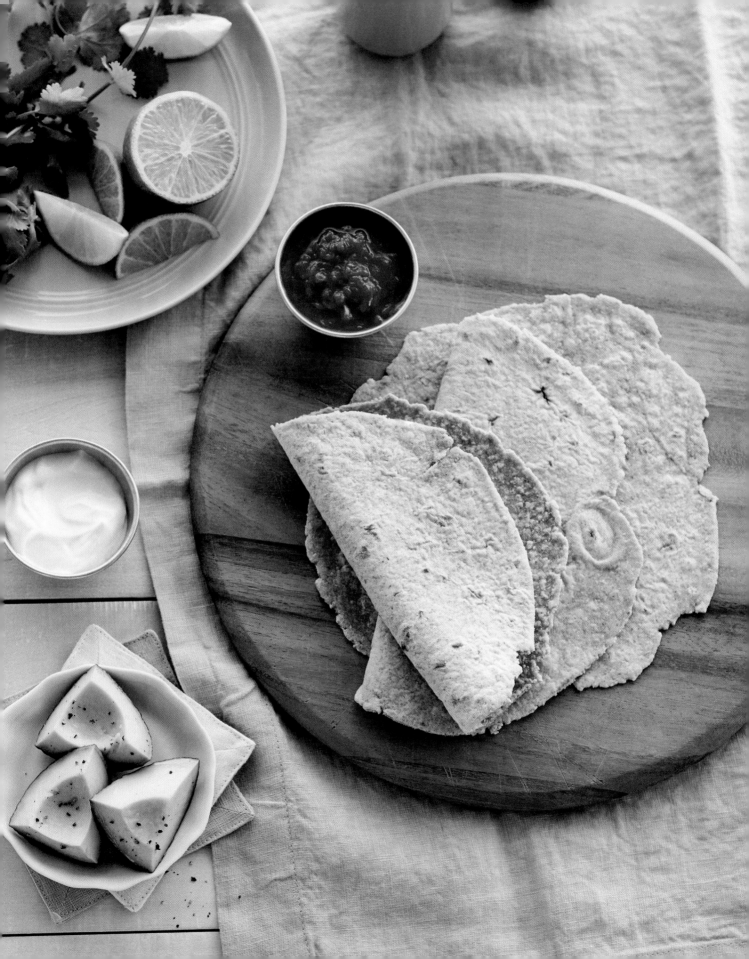

Multigrain Buns

These buns are so light and soft you would never believe there are ancient grains in them. Teff, buckwheat and chia are incognito but make these buns perfect for sandwiches, burgers or anything that requires a hardy bun. Even gluten-eaters won't be able to tell the difference!

MAKES SIXTEEN 3 1/2-INCH (9 CM) BUNS OR 8 MINI-SUBMARINE SANDWICH BUNS

1 cup (250 mL) teff flour

¾ cup (175 mL) light buckwheat flour

¾ cup (175 mL) tapioca starch

⅓ cup (75 mL) ground chia seeds

3 Tbsp (45 mL) psyllium husks

2 tsp (10 mL) xanthan gum

1 Tbsp (15 mL) quick-rising yeast

2 Tbsp (30 mL) organic cane sugar

1 ½ tsp (7 mL) salt

½ tsp (2 mL) cream of tartar

1 ½ cups (375 mL) warm water at 120–125°F (50–52°C)

2 large eggs

2 Tbsp (30 mL) grapeseed oil, plus oil for hands

1 Tbsp (15 mL) fancy molasses

1 tsp (5 mL) apple cider vinegar

⅓ cup (75 mL) raw, unsalted sunflower seeds

2 Tbsp (30 mL) large-flake oats

Line a large baking sheet with parchment paper.

Mix the teff and buckwheat flours, tapioca starch, chia, psyllium, xanthan gum, yeast, sugar, salt and cream of tartar in the bowl of a stand mixer using the paddle attachment, or use a large bowl and a handheld mixer. Stir in the warm water until evenly combined. Add the eggs, oil, molasses and vinegar. Work ¼ cup (60 mL) of the sunflower seeds into the dough. Mix for 5 minutes.

Lightly oil the inside of a ¼ cup (60 mL) measure. Oil your hands and measure ¼ cup (60 mL) of dough into the palm of your hand. Roll the dough into a ball and place it on the parchment. Lightly flatten to about 1 inch (2.5 cm) thickness. Sprinkle each dough ball with a few oats and the remaining sunflower seeds. Place the baking sheet in a warm, draft-free area, covered with a dry towel, until dough balls have doubled in size, 40 minutes to 1 hour.

Preheat the oven to 350°F (180°C).

Bake the buns for 19 to 21 minutes, until golden. Remove the buns from the oven and let rest on the baking sheet for 10 minutes before serving.

PER SERVING: Energy 140 calories; Protein 4 g; Carbohydrates 22 g; Dietary Fiber 5 g; Fat 4.5 g; Sugar 3 g; Cholesterol 25 mg; Sodium 190 mg

STORAGE

Room Temperature: airtight container or bag, 4 days

Refrigerator: airtight container or bag, 5 days

Freezer: airtight freezer bag or container, 1 month

BAKING TIP

For mini-submarine buns, use a lightly greased
½ cup (125 mL) measure to scoop the dough into your oiled
hands. Roll out to a 1 ¼- to 1 ½-inch (3—4 cm) wide log.
Make three evenly spaced, shallow diagonal slits in the top of the
dough. Cover the buns with a dry dish towel and let rise in a warm,
draft-free spot until doubled in size, 45 minutes to 1 hour.
Bake at 350°F (180°C) for 19 to 21 minutes, until golden.

White Dinner Buns

These buns are great for any large family brunch or dinner, or as a staple to have ready for lunches and sandwiches throughout the week. Easily baked in a standard muffin tin, these beauties are golden and crusty on the outside and fluffy and moist on the inside. Sorghum and chia help to beef up the nutrients, making these a healthier option than any regular white bun!

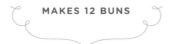

MAKES 12 BUNS

1 cup (250 mL) sorghum flour

¾ cup (175 mL) sweet rice flour

¾ cup (175 mL) tapioca starch

⅓ cup (75 mL) ground chia seeds

3 Tbsp (45 mL) psyllium husks

1 tsp (5 mL) xanthan gum

2 Tbsp (30 mL) organic
    cane sugar

1 Tbsp (15 mL) quick-rising yeast

1 ½ tsp (7 mL) salt

½ tsp (2 mL) cream of tartar

1 ½ cups (375 mL) warm 1% milk
    or milk substitute at 120–125°F
    (50–52°C)

2 large eggs

2 Tbsp (30 mL) grapeseed
    or organic light-tasting oil

1 tsp (5 mL) apple cider vinegar

Lightly grease a standard 12-cup muffin tin.

Place the sorghum and rice flours, tapioca starch, chia, psyllium, xanthan gum, sugar, yeast, salt and cream of tartar in the bowl of a stand mixer or large bowl. Stir all the ingredients together using a paddle attachment or whisk. Pour in the warm milk and mix with the paddle attachment or a handheld mixer on low speed until combined. Add the eggs, oil and apple cider vinegar. Mix on medium speed for 3 to 4 minutes. Flour your hands. Scoop out ⅓ cup (75 mL) of dough and roll it into a ball. Place each ball in a muffin cup. Cover the entire pan with a dry dish towel and place it in a warm, draft-free area to rise until balls are doubled in size, 40 minutes to 1 hour.

Preheat the oven to 350°F (180°C).

Bake the buns for 20 to 25 minutes, or until an instant read thermometer inserted in the center of one reads 200°F (100°C). Place aluminum foil over the buns halfway through the baking process, when they are perfectly golden, to prevent overbrowning. Remove from the oven and carefully transfer the buns to a cooling rack to prevent them from getting soggy.

PER SERVING: Energy 190 calories; Protein 5 g; Carbohydrates 30 g; Dietary Fiber 5 g; Fat 5 g; Sugar 4 g; Cholesterol 35 mg; Sodium 215 mg

STORAGE

Room Temperature: airtight container or bag, 4 days

Refrigerator: airtight container or bag, 4 days

Freezer: airtight freezer bag or container, 2 weeks

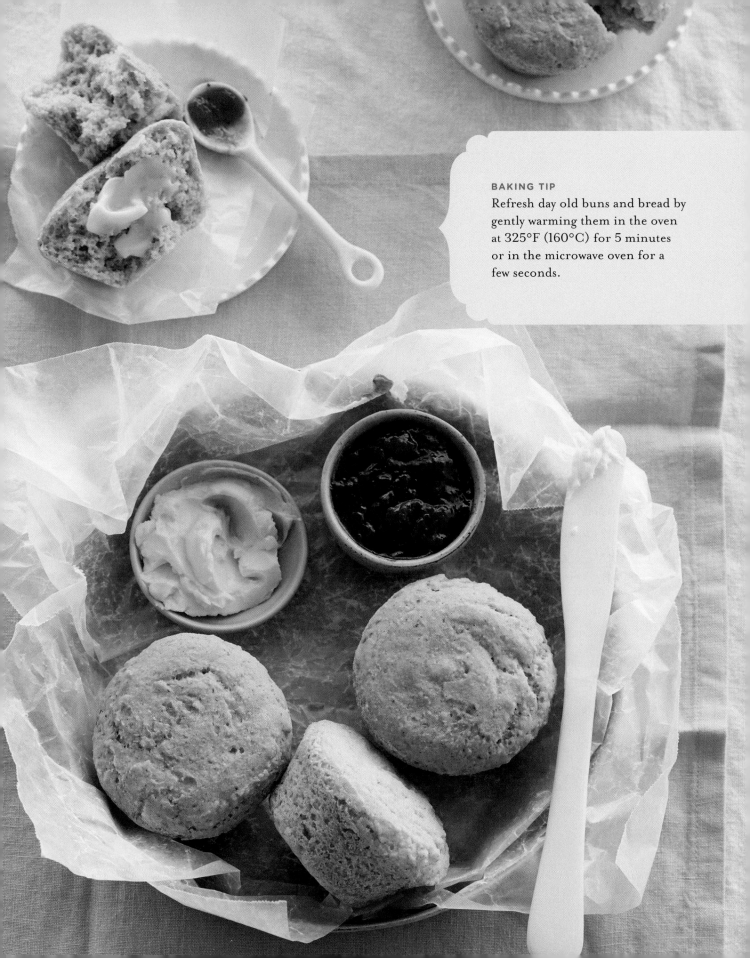

BAKING TIP
Refresh day old buns and bread by gently warming them in the oven at 325°F (160°C) for 5 minutes or in the microwave oven for a few seconds.

Homemade Soft Pretzels

Chewy homemade pretzels with coarse salt are a family favorite of ours.
Ready to dip in your favorite pizza or cheese sauce, this gluten-free version
is made with sorghum and rice flours.

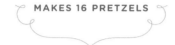

MAKES 16 PRETZELS

1 cup (250 mL) sweet rice flour

²/₃ cup (150 mL) sorghum flour

½ cup (125 mL) brown rice flour

2 Tbsp (30 mL) psyllium husks

1 Tbsp (15 mL) quick-rising yeast

2 tsp (10 mL) organic cane sugar

1 tsp (5 mL) xanthan gum

¼ tsp (1 mL) salt

1 cup + 2 Tbsp (280 mL) warm
   water at 120–125°F (50–52°C)

2 Tbsp (30 mL) grapeseed or
   organic light-tasting oil (plus
   oil for rolling and brushing)

¼ tsp (1 mL) coarse salt

Line a large baking sheet with parchment paper.

Whisk the sweet rice, sorghum and brown rice flours, psyllium, yeast, sugar, xanthan gum and salt in a stand mixer, or whisk in a medium bowl. Stir in the warm water and oil until incorporated. Use the paddle attachment on medium speed to mix the dough or hand-knead the dough for about 5 minutes. Roll the dough into a log, cut it into 16 equal pieces and cover with a slightly damp cloth or plastic wrap.

Oil your hands and roll one piece of dough into a 7- or 8-inch (18–20 cm) long rope. Form a U-shape, then cross both ends over the top of each other, bringing each one to the opposite side of the circle to form a pretzel shape. Place on the baking sheet, brush with a slight touch of oil, sprinkle with coarse salt and cover with a towel. Repeat with the remaining dough. Let the pretzels rise, covered, in a warm draft-free place until doubled in size (45 minutes to 1 hour).

Preheat the oven to 375°F (190°C).

Bake the pretzels for 20 minutes until golden brown. Serve warm.

PER SERVING: Energy 90 calories; Protein 2 g; Carbohydrates 16 g; Dietary Fiber 2 g; Fat 2 g; Sugar 1 g; Cholesterol 0 mg; Sodium 65 mg

STORAGE

Refrigerator: airtight container or bag, 1 day

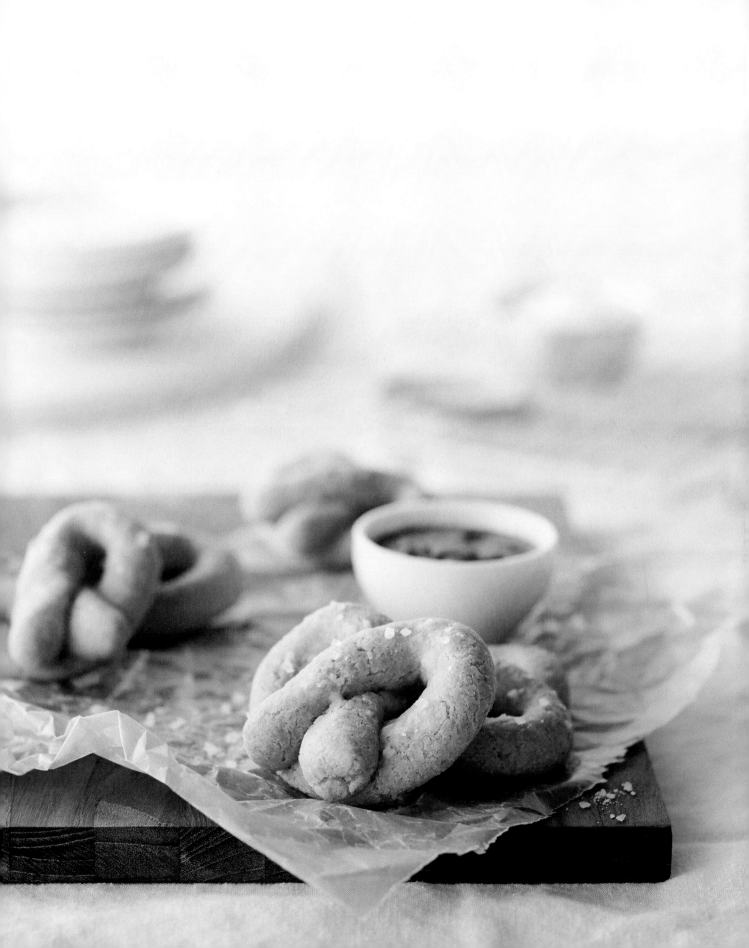

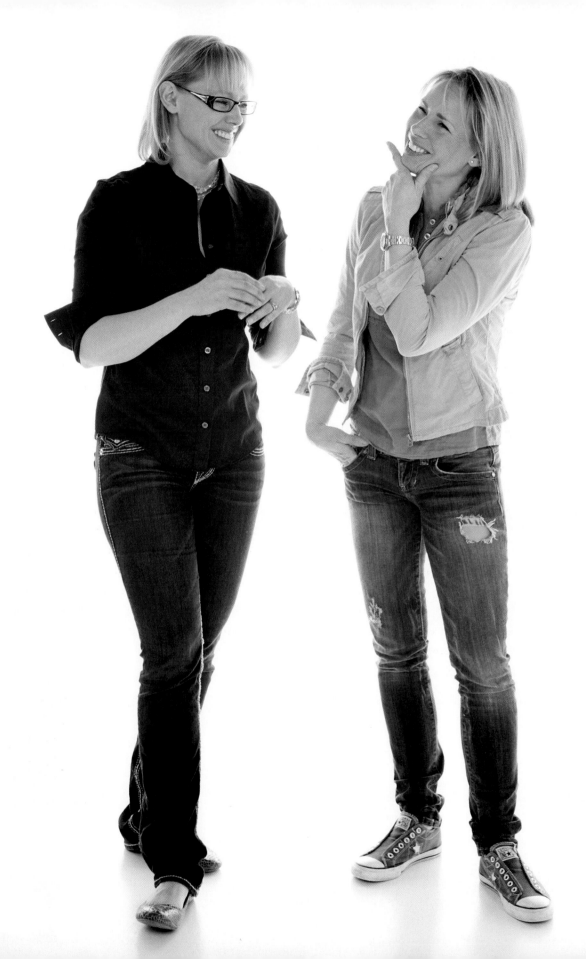

Acknowledgments

We are tremendously fortunate to have Ian, Paul, Sydney, Alyssa and Aston as never-ending sources of inspiration, creative ideas and honesty about our cooking. We owe a great deal of thanks to our late father, Swen Runkvist, who was very proud of his daughters and could talk about us all day. If you were ever one of those people he spoke to (including all of his dear friends), thanks for listening!

We are grateful for the constant support of Vera Friesen, Bill and Val Green, Dallas Green, Bobbi and Ashley Beuker, Jeff and Joanne Blake, Kate Blake and Jason Currier, Marg and Tony Blake and the entire Barber clan in England. We appreciate the inspiration and support from all of our seriously amazing and wonderful extended family, the Arps, the Runkvists, the Deasons and the late Ray and Joy Hemming.

We will always be touched by and grateful for the support and teachings of our late grandparents, Esther, George and Florence, and even our great-grandparents who paved the way for us, working their butts off immigrating to Canada from Europe with very little and fearlessly making a new start, farming in the not-always-kind prairies. They helped to define that ol' intrepid farmer attitude of finding a way regardless of skills and circumstances. Thank you to them for cherishing and mastering home baking with natural, whole foods and grains, long before major food processing came into the world. Grandma's kitchen was an inspiring place, always dusted with flour and smelling of apples, coffee and boiling potatoes.

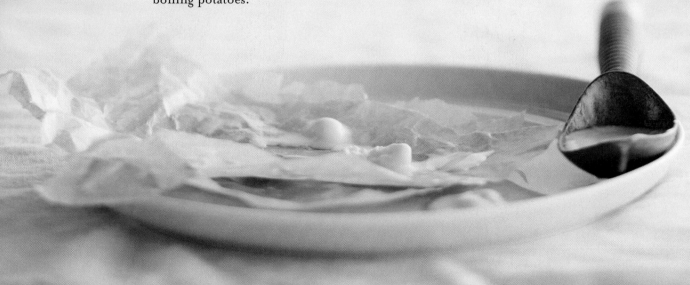

We always thank our numerous industry advisors and supporters who continue to answer our urgent, often complex questions and take our last-minute calls without fail. Sergio Nuñez de Arco, Marcos Guevara, Laurie Scanlin and Claire Burnett, Bob Moore, Nancy Garner, Sarah House and the entire, incredibly cool Bob's Red Mill team, Jeffrey and Amy Barnes at Edison Grainery, George Aramayo at Arrow Foods, Francisco Diez-Canseco and Magdalena Diez-Canseco. Thank you to all of our dear friends for the continued cheers and consulting and for allowing us to feed you our recipes "in development": Alicia Colgan, Terri Reagan, Treena Klagenberg and Rob Person, Sandy Wasylyniuk, Sandy Blydo, Christina Lewis, Jake and Tara Trottier, Karen and James Johnston, Rusty Livingston and Jeff Knisely, Steve Arnott and Onalee Orchard, Mia and Ian Kruger, Sara Busby, Kerri Rosenbaum Barr, Billijon Morgan, Ken and Noreen McLean and Sheila, Mark and Jessie Gordon, Dr. Stephanie Anisko, Jocelyn Campanaro and Craig Billington, Stefani Farkas, Frank Dyson, Kathy and John Holford, Rose Gage and Eddy Smith, Linda Beaudoin, Colin and Amanda Gillan, Nella Mirante, Gordon Kirke, Stan Butler, Theresa Nesbitt, Elfreda Pretorius, the Addersons, Coralee Burnett, Shaundra Carvey-Parker, Heather Dyer, Shela Shapiro, Leslie Edmunds, Janine Kemp, Ashley Whitenect, Nicki and Chad Hayden, Ken and Mary Kruger, Terry Paluszkiewicz and Annica Sjoberg.

We always, always, always thank independent, hardworking farmers EVERYWHERE. They never seem to expect any thanks, but they keep working hard to put food on our tables. We love hearing that we are helping to positively affect them by spreading the word about ancient grains. Farmers feed cities. Bless those farmers!

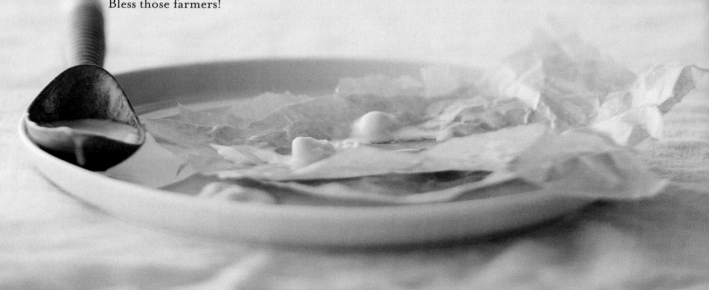

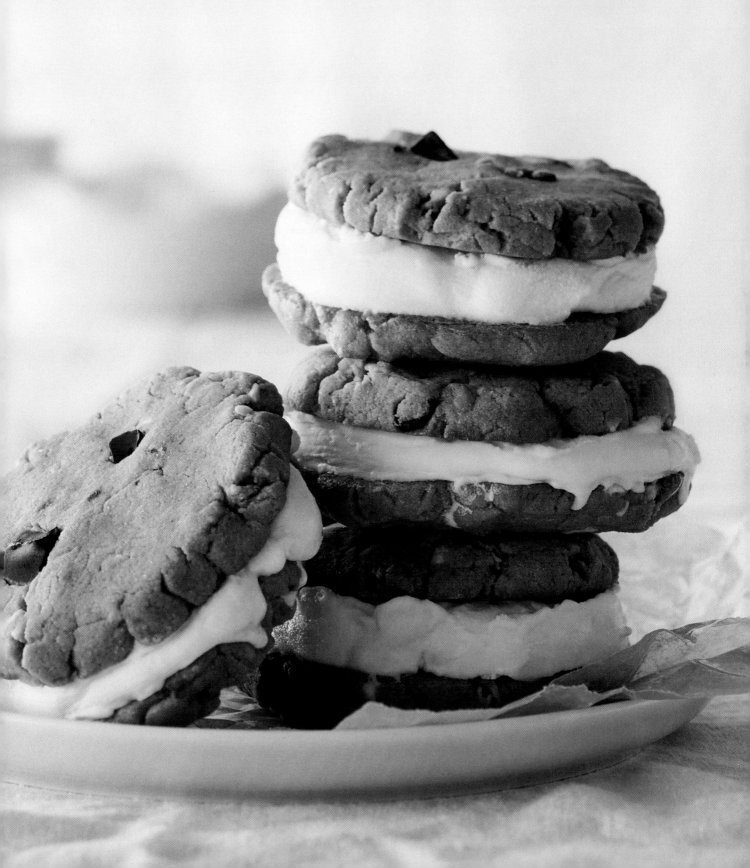

Popular Gluten-Free Ingredients

Here is our list of popular gluten-free seeds, grains, flours and starches you can find in stores today. Ingredients used in this book are highlighted in yellow.

INGREDIENT	ORIGIN	FLAVOR	PROPERTIES	TIPS
ALMOND FLOUR	Nut	Sweet, made of ground blanched almonds, subtle, nutty	Dense, finer grind than meal	Not great for high heat, possible substitute for oat flour in baking
ALMOND MEAL	Nut	Made of ground almonds, sweet, subtle, nutty	Coarse, dense, chewier baking	Not great for high heat, possible substitute for oatmeal in baking
AMARANTH FLOUR	Seed (non-grass)	Sweet, malty, herbaceous, distinctive/dominant	Baking browns quickly, gelatinous	High glycemic, may be bitter
ARROWROOT FLOUR (STARCH)	Root	Smells slightly like anise, but bakes neutral	Absorbs more liquid than other starches, easy to digest	Best substitute for tapioca starch
BROWN RICE FLOUR	Grain (cereal, grass)	Neutral, bland, slightly nutty	Grainy, coarse texture, adds fiber	Store in refrigerator; use with protein-rich flours for better structure; can be used to thicken, especially in frozen or refrigerated recipes to prevent separation of liquids; not to be confused with sweet rice flour or rice starch
BUCKWHEAT FLOUR (DARK)	Seed (non-grass)	Stronger nutty, earthy flavor than light	High fiber, whole wheat appearance	Store in refrigerator, use in recipes where color is not noticeable
BUCKWHEAT FLOUR (LIGHT)	Seed (non-grass)	Milder, more neutral than dark buckwheat, nutty, earthy	High fiber, whole wheat appearance	Store in refrigerator, light is best for baking
CHESTNUT FLOUR	Nut	Made with ground chestnuts, earthy, nutty, sweet	Fibrous texture	Combine with protein-rich flour for structure
CHIA, GROUND	Seed (non-grass)	Mild, neutral	Gelatinous, binding properties	Omega-3 rich, seedy texture, can replace a portion of some fats (butter, egg) in baking

INGREDIENT	ORIGIN	FLAVOR	PROPERTIES	TIPS
CHICKPEA FLOUR	Bean/legume	Sweet, rich, stronger taste than rice flour	Fine texture	High in protein, lower carbohydrate option
COCONUT FLOUR	**Nut**	**Coconut fragrance, sweet**	**Can be drying, may use extra egg to lighten, soaks up moisture, can make baking dense**	**Safe at high temperatures, high fiber, lower-carbohydrate option**
CORNMEAL	**Grain (cereal, grass)**	**Nutty, coarse**	**Fibrous, may make baking dense, gritty**	**Good for breading and specific cakes and biscuits**
CORNSTARCH	**Starch, grain (cereal, grass)**	**Flavorless, neutral**	**A light starch, lightens and adds air, improves crispness, bonds the lightest of all starches**	**Closest substitute for potato or tapioca starch, speeds rising with yeast, may substitute with arrowroot starch**
FAVA BEAN FLOUR	Bean/legume	Earthy, bean flavor	Creamy color, high fiber	Brown rice substitute
FLAX, GROUND	Seed (non-grass)	Gritty, earthy, nutty	Seedy appearance, binding properties	Omega-3 rich, goes rancid quickly, refrigerate
GARFAVA FLOUR	Bean/legume	Distinct bean flavor	A mixture of garbanzo, (chickpea) fava and Romano beans	Good used as part of blend in doughs and cakes, best used with other dominant flavors
GUAR GUM	Gum, bean/legume	Bland, neutral	A stabilizer, improves thickening, improves rising, resilience	Light colored, a stronger binder useful in doughs and yeast breads, alternative to xanthan gum
HAZELNUT FLOUR	**Nut**	**Hazelnut aroma, sweet, nutty, rich flavor**	**Adds a richer flavor, texture more grainy**	**Lower-carbohydrate choice, keep refrigerated**
HEMP FLOUR	Seed (non-grass)	Earthy, nutty, gritty	High fiber	Protein-rich, unpleasant dominant taste if overused
KANIWA FLOUR	Seed (non-grass)	Sweeter, milder and more neutral than quinoa, grainy, nutty, earthy	Protein-rich, can replace bread crumbs	Flavor may overpower if overused
MESQUITE FLOUR	Seed (non-grass)	Molasses-like flavor, earthy, sweet, may get stronger with cooking	Dark, whole grain appearance	Distinctive taste may dominate
MILLET FLOUR	**Seed (non-grass)**	**Light, mild, neutral, nutty, dusty, sweet**	**Lightens baked goods, yellow/creamy color, adds structure**	**Good for yeast breads, doughs and flatbreads**
MONTINA FLOUR (INDIAN RICE GRASS)	Grain (cereal, grass)	Wheat-like in taste and texture	Whole wheat–like appearance	Not related to rice, flavor may overpower, best in darker baking

Continued

Popular Gluten-Free Ingredients (continued)

INGREDIENT	ORIGIN	FLAVOR	PROPERTIES	TIPS
OAT FLOUR	**Grain (cereal, grass)**	**Light, mild, neutral, slightly sweet, not dominant**	**Ground oatmeal (flakes) adds structure**	**Highly versatile, mild binding properties, great for most quick breads**
PEANUT FLOUR	Nut	Peanut taste	Soaks up moisture, can be drying, peanut flavor noticeable	Some flours are defatted (partially), may be roasted light, medium or dark
PEA PROTEIN (FLOUR)	Bean/legume	Earthy, starchy	Green color apparent	Don't use where color is not desired
POTATO FLOUR	Root	Potato flavor	Made of dried ground potatoes, absorbs liquid well, dense (heavier than rice flour), makes chewier, softer	Works well with rice flour, can be replaced with xanthan or guar gum in some cases, overuse can have gummy result
POTATO STARCH	Root	Flavorless	Moderate binding ability, chewier, helps rising, lightens, makes chewier	Best used along with tapioca starch or cornstarch, no significant nutrition
PSYLLIUM HUSKS	**Seed (non-grass)**	**No flavor**	**Binds moisture, makes baking less crumbly**	**High fiber, promotes digestion**
QUINOA FLOUR	**Seed (non-grass)**	**Nutty, delicate**	**Versatile, dense flour**	**Overuse in a blend may overpower flavor, high nutrition, great for most quick breads**
RICE STARCH	Grain (cereal, grass)	Similar to sweet rice flour	Improves chewiness, a heavier starch, thickening agent	Can be grainy, not to be confused with rice flour
SORGHUM FLOUR	**Grain (cereal, grass)**	**Wheat-like flavor, sweet, neutral, dusty**	**Dull color, superfine texture**	**Promotes digestion, whole wheat–like texture and color, great for most quick breads**
SOYBEAN (SOY) FLOUR	Bean/legume	Stronger flavor than rice flour, earthy	Fine texture	Lower carbohydrate option, fibrous
SWEET POTATO FLOUR	Root	Sweet	Yellow color, improves chewiness, browning	Overuse can be gummy

INGREDIENT	ORIGIN	FLAVOR	PROPERTIES	TIPS
SWEET RICE FLOUR	Seed (non-grass)	Starchy, bland, neutral	Light flour, thickening agent	AKA glutinous rice flour (sticky rice flour), thickens
TAPIOCA STARCH (FLOUR)	Root	Neutral, tasteless	Holds stronger than other starches, lightens, improves rising, improves browning, makes chewier	Speeds rising with yeast, closest substitute is cornstarch, AKA cassava or yucca, overuse will be gummy
TEFF FLOUR	Grain (cereal, grass)	Slightly sour taste, nutty, hazelnut flavor (lighter colored teff), molasses flavor (darker colored teff)	Gelatinous	Flavor may overpower, works well in quick breads
WHITE RICE FLOUR	Grain (cereal, grass)	Bland, neutral	Simple to work with, sometimes grainy	Easy to find, use with protein-rich flours for better structure, not to be confused with sweet rice flour or rice starch, no real nutrition
WILD RICE FLOUR	Grain (cereal, grass)	Hardy, earthy	Dark color, great in pastries and quick breads	Not the same as other rice products, has long shelf-life, distinctive flavor may overpower
XANTHAN GUM	Gum (corn), grain (cereal, grass)	Flavorless	A stabilizer, improves rising and thickening, forms a gel in water, helps starches to combine, baked goods have a lighter texture	Originates from dairy, wheat or soy; no nutritional value; a stronger binder useful in doughs and yeast breads; substitutes are flax, psyllium, chia and eggs; ensure purchase gluten-free if required

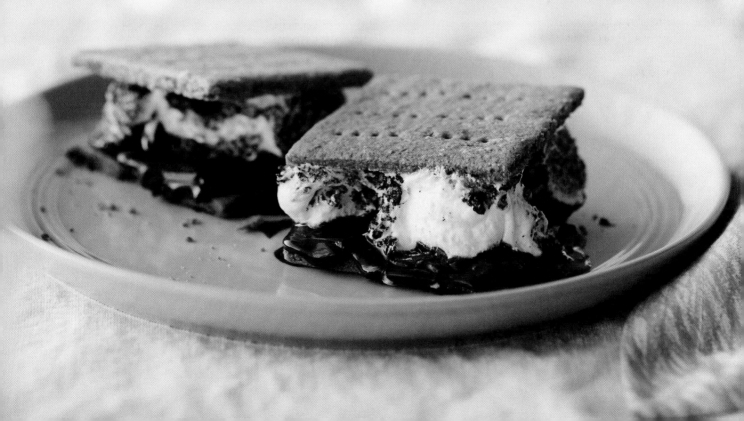

Gluten-Free Ingredients and Basic Nutritional Values: Quick Reference Table

INGREDIENT (30 G SERVING)	CALORIES	PROTEIN (G)	CARBS (G)	FIBER (G)	FAT (G)	SUGAR (G)	CHOLESTEROL (MG)	SODIUM (MG)	COMPLETE PROTEIN
Almond flour	170	6	6	3	15	1	0	10	N
Almond meal	170	6	6	3	15	1	0	10	N
Amaranth flour	110	4	20	3	2	0	0	5	N
Arrowroot starch (flour)	110	0	26	1	0	0	0	0	N
Brown rice flour	110	2	23	1	1	0	0	0	N
Buckwheat flour (dark)	113	4	21	4	1	0	0	0	Y
Buckwheat flour (light)	110	4	25	2	0.5	0	0	0	Y
Chestnut flour	120	2	24	3	1	6	0	6	Y
Chia, ground	150	5	13	10	9	0	0	0	Y
Chickpea flour	110	6	18	5	2	3	0	5	N
Coconut flour	130	4	17	11	4.5	0	0	65	N
Cornmeal (yellow)	110	2	23	2	1	0	0	10	N
Cornstarch	110	0	27	0	0	0	0	0	N
Fava bean flour	108	8	18	7	0	0.5	0	0	N
Flax, ground	170	6	9	6	13	0	0	0	Y
Garfava flour	110	6	18	6	1.5	3	0	5	N
Guar gum	90	0	26	26	0	0	0	10	N
Hazelnut flour	180	4	5	3	17	1	0	0	N
Hemp flour	100	12	8	6	3	0	0	0	Y
Kaniwa flour*	120	6	19	2	2.5	0	0	0	Y
Mesquite flour*	136	4	30	12	1	20	0	0	Y

INGREDIENT (30 G SERVING)	CALORIES	PROTEIN (G)	CARBS (G)	FIBER (G)	FAT (G)	SUGAR (G)	CHOLESTEROL (MG)	SODIUM (MG)	COMPLETE PROTEIN
Millet flour	110	3	22	4	1	0	0	0	N
Montina flour*	125	5	22	8	1	0	0	0	N
Oat flour	110	4	18	3	2	0	0	0	N
Peanut flour* (low fat/partially defatted)	110	14	9	4	4	0	0	0	N
Peanut flour* (defatted)	98	15	10	5	0	2.5	0	54	N
Pea protein* (flour)	118	22	1	0	2	0	0	320	N
Potato flour*	110	3	24	2	0	0	0	10	N
Potato starch	100	0	25	0	0	0	0	0	N
Psyllium husks*	17	2	0	24	0	0	0	23	N
Quinoa flour	130	4	22	4	2	0	0	10	Y
Quinoa seeds	133	5	23	3	2	1	0	8	Y
Rice starch*	110	0	30	0	0	0	0	0	N
Sorghum flour	110	2	23	2	1	1	0	0	N
Soybean (soy) flour	122	11	9	4	7	3	0	0	Y
Sweet rice flour	110	2	24	1	0	1	0	0	N
Tapioca starch (flour)	100	0	26	0	0	0	0	0	N
Teff flour	110	4	22	4	1	0	0	0	Y
White rice flour	110	2	24	1	0	0	0	0	N
Xanthan gum	35	0	27	27	0	0	0	35	N

*Values are approximate

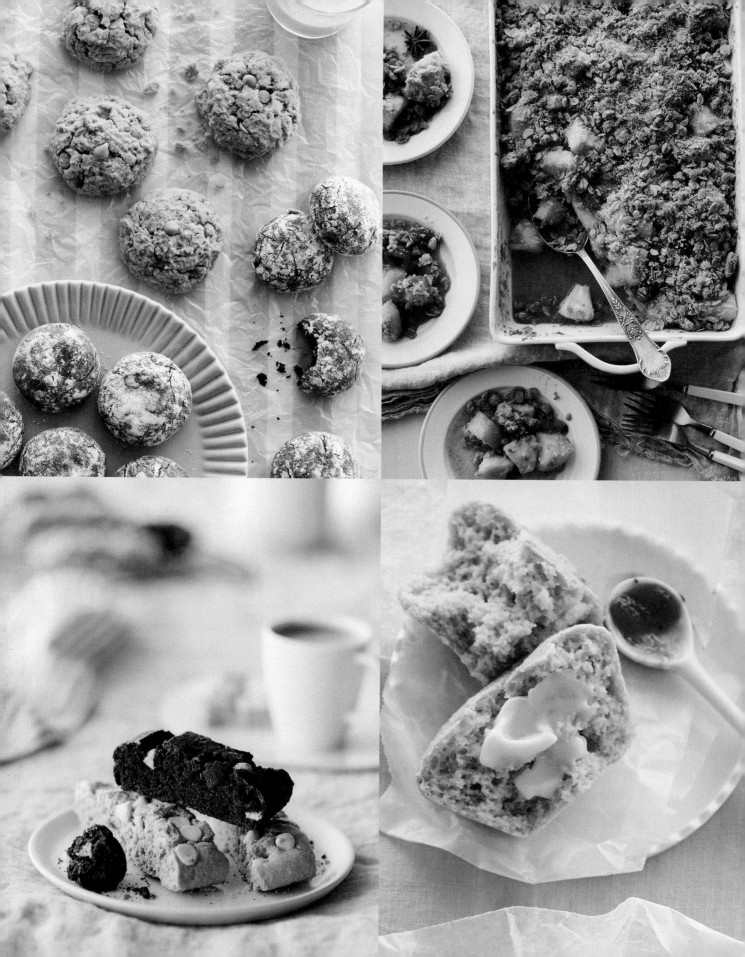

References

Gomez, M., Talegon, M. & la Hera, E. 2013. Influence of mixing on quality of gluten-free bread. *Journal of Food Quality*, 36(2): 139-145.

Green, P., & Hemming, C. 2012. Introduction: Revolutionizing health and fitness with quinoa. *Quinoa Revolution*; xiii.

Wieser, H. 2007. Chemistry of gluten proteins. *Food Microbiology*, 24(2): 115-119.

Wieser, H. 1996. Relation between gliadin structure and coeliac toxicity. *Acta Paediatr Suppl.*, 4(12): 3-9.

Wieser, H. 1995. The precipitating factor in coeliac disease. *Baillieres Clin Gastroenterol*, 9(20): 191-207.

Index

A

agar agar, binder xxxv

agave xxxix

almond, Cherry Almond
Truffles 154
Cranberry Almond
Energy Bites 26

Almond Ancient Grain
Cupcakes 63

almond flour xxi, xxii,
188, 192

almond meal 188, 192

almond milk xlii

altitude, effect xlvii

amaranth *flakes, flour, puffs, seeds*
xxi, xxii, xxvii, 188, 192

Ancient Grain Angel Food
Cake 81

Ancient Grain Bread 169

Ancient Grain Pound Cake 80

Ancient Grain Summer Fruit
Tarts 139

Ancient Grain Tortilla
Wraps 176

ancient grains, *benefits* xiii, xviii

angel food cake, Ancient
Grain 81

apple, Baked Apple Crumble
with Carrot and Raisin
Spice Filling 142
Caramel Apple Tarte
Tatin 111
Cinnamon Apple
Coffee Cake 83

Apple Raisin Oat Squares 30

apricot, Carrot Apricot
Squares 27

Apricot, Walnut and Pine Nut
Granola Bars 29

arrowroot starch (flour) xxi,
xxii, 188, 192

B

bacon, Toffee Maple Bacon
Scones 56

Baked Apple Crumble with
Carrot and Raisin Spice
Filling 142

baking powder, leavening
agent xxxvii

baking soda, leavening
agent xxxvii

banana, Chocolate Swirl
Banana Loaf 73

Banana Breakfast Bread 70

bark, Candied Ginger Orange
and Pistachio Bark 153
Thai Coconut Dark
Chocolate Bark with
Lime Zest 152

bars, Apricot, Walnut and
Pine Nut Granola Bars 29
Espresso Cookie Bars with
Honey Marshmallow
Meringue 38

Basil Pesto and Pine Nut
Loaf 173

beets, Honey-Roasted Beet
and Lemon Cheesecake 140

berries, see *blackberries*
see *blueberries*
see *raspberries*
see *strawberries*
Wild Berry Pie 114

binders and stabilizers xxxiv,
xxxvi

biscotti, Citrus Sorghum
and Oat Biscotti 24
Double Chocolate Sorghum
and Teff Biscotti 23

biscuits, Golden Buttermilk
Biscuits 54

Mint Cherry Country
    Baked Biscuits 51
Parmesan Salt and Pepper
    Biscuits 55
Blackberry Honey Clafoutis 94
blondies, Milk Chocolate
    and Orange Blondies 39
Praline Cheesecake
    Blondies 40
blueberries, Blueberry Goat
    Cheese Tart 116
Mashed Blueberry Lime
    Hand Pies 112
Wild Blueberry Buttermilk
    Bran Muffins 61
bread, Ancient Grain
    Bread 169
Chipotle Cheddar Quick
    Bread 172
Dill Cilantro Buttermilk
    Bread with Mint 167
Enriched White Bread 162
French Bread 164
Molasses Ancient Grain
    Loaf 170
Tender Egg Bread
    (Challah) 166
Breakfast Popover Loaf 71
brown rice flour xxi, xxii,
    188, 192
brown sugar, sweeteners xxxix
brownies, Chocolate Hazelnut
    Brownies 41
buckwheat, light, dark, flour, groats,
    flakes xxi, xxii, 188, 192
buns, Multigrain Buns 178
    White Dinner Buns 180
butter, fats in baking xlii
butter, nuts xlii
buttermilk xlii
buttermilk recipes, Dill
    Cilantro Buttermilk
    Bread with Mint 167
Golden Buttermilk
    Biscuits 54

Wild Blueberry Buttermilk
    Bran Muffins 61
butterscotch, Carrot
    Butterscotch Cookies 4

C
cakes 43
Candied Ginger, Orange
    and Pistachio Bark 153
cane sugar, organic xxxix, xl
caramel, Salted Caramel Pecan
    Shortbread Bites 17
Praline Cheesecake
    Blondies 40
Caramel Apple Tarte
    Tatin 111
carrot, Baked Apple Crumble
    with Carrot and Raisin
    Spice Filling 142
Honey Ginger Carrot Cakes
    with Lime Cream Cheese
    Frosting 64
Carrot Apricot Squares 27
Carrot Butterscotch Cookies 4
Carrot Spice Pie 118
challah, Tender Egg Bread 166
cheese, Cheddar, Chipotle
    Cheddar Quick Bread 172
    cream cheese, Oat, Strawberry
    and Cream Cheese
    Thumbprint Cookies 7
Chocolate Cream Cheese
    Coconut Cake 88
Cream Cheese Pastry 104
    goat cheese, Blueberry Goat
    Cheese Tart 116
cheesecake, Honey-
    Roasted Beet and Lemon
    Cheesecake 140
Mini Maple Cherry
    Cheesecakes 79
Praline Cheesecake
    Blondies 40

cherry, Mint Cherry Country
    Baked Biscuits 51
Mini Maple Cherry
    Cheesecakes 79
Cherry Almond Truffles 154
chestnut flour 188, 192
Chewy Raisin Oatmeal
    Chia Cookies 6
chia, binder xxxiv, xxxv, xxxvi
chia, seeds xxxiii, xliii, xlvi,
    188, 192
chickpea flour xxi, 188, 192
Chipotle Cheddar Quick
    Bread 172
Chocolate Cream Cheese
    Coconut Cake 88
Chocolate Fruit and Nut
    Chia Squares 34
Chocolate Hazelnut
    Brownies 41
Chocolate Quinoa Pie 122
Chocolate Swirl Banana
    Loaf 73
Chocolate, Walnut and Prune
    Millet Quinoa Squares 35
Chocolate Whirl Cookies 9
Chocolate Whoopie Pies 21
cinnamon, Maple Raisin
    Cinnamon Buns 74
Cinnamon Apple Coffee
    Cake 83
clafoutis, Blackberry Honey 94
coconut, Chocolate Cream
    Cheese Coconut Cake 88
Chocolate Fruit and Nut
    Chia Squares 34
Hawaiian Oat Squares 31
Strawberry and Raspberry
    Coconut Cream
    Trifle 146
Thai Coconut Dark
    Chocolate Bark with
    Lime Zest 152
Triple Chocolate Coconut
    Chia Cookies 16

coconut flour xxi, xxiii, 189, 192
coconut milk xlii
coconut oil xlii, xliii
coconut sugar xxxix, xl
Coconut Cake with Whipped Yogurt Frosting 84
coffee cake, Cinnamon Apple 83
coffee grinder, use of xliv
cookies 1
cornmeal 189, 192
cornstarch xxi, xxiii, 189, 192
Cranberry Almond Energy Bites 26
Cranberry Lemon Millet Quinoa Squares 36
Cranberry Lemon Oatcakes 50
Cranberry Walnut and Rosemary Muffins 58
Cream Cheese Pastry 104
cream of tartar xxxvii
crepes, Lemon Crepe Cake 86
cupcakes, Almond Ancient Grain Cupcakes 63

D
dairy xlii
dairy-free, alternatives xlii
dates, Cherry Almond Truffles 154
   Pecan Date Pie 120
Demerara sugar xxxix, xl
Devil's Food Cake 90
Dill Cilantro Buttermilk Bread with Mint 167
Double-Layer Chocolate Chia Zucchini Cake 138
doughnuts, Double Chocolate Cake Doughnuts 68
   Old-Fashioned Cake Doughnuts 67

E
eggs, binder xxxiv, xxxv, xxxvi
   use in baking xlii, xlvi
   substitutes xliii
Enriched White Bread 162
equipment, baking xliii, xlvii
Espresso Cookie Bars with Honey Marshmallow Meringue 38

F
fats, use in baking xlii
favabean flour 189, 192
fig, Oat Fig Newtons 18
flakes, *ancient grain,* Cherry Almond Truffles 154
   Chocolate Fruit and Nut Chia Squares 34
   Cranberry Almond Energy Bites 26
   Mint Matcha Morsels 22
flax xxxiv, xxxv, xxxvi, xliii, 189, 192
flour, blends xxvi
flour, gluten-free xxi
flour, grinding xxviii, xxix
flour, sprouted grains xxi
flour, storage xxi
flour, weighing and measuring xxx
Fluffy White Quinoa Cake 82
French Bread 164

G
garbanzo flour, *see chickpea*
garfava flour xxi, 189, 192
gelatin, binder xxxv
genetic modification xi
ginger, Candied Ginger, Orange and Pistachio Bark 153
   Honey Ginger Carrot Cakes with Lime Cream Cheese Frosting 64

Gingerbread Cookies 137
Ginger Squash Molasses Cookies 15
gluten, contamination xii, xiii
gluten proteins xviii
gluten-free, benefits xi, xlvii, xlviii, xlix, xlx, li
gluten-free, conventional products x
gluten-free, flours and starches xx, xxi
gluten-free, health and nutrition xi, xii, xviii, xlviii, xlix, xlx, li
gluten-free, ingredients xiv
gluten-free, labeling xii
gluten-free, weight loss xlx, li
gluten-free, where to purchase xiii
Gluten-Free Pie Pastry I 102
Gluten-Free Pie Pastry II 103
Golden Buttermilk Biscuits 54
Graham Peanut Butter Chocolate Bites 156
Graham-Style Wafer Crumb Crust 108
Graham-Style Wafers 46
granola bars, Apricot, Walnut and Pine Nut 29
grapeseed oil xlii
grinding flour xxviii, xxix, xliv
guar gum, binder xxxiv, xxxv, xlvi, 189, 192

H
Hawaiian Oat Squares 31
hazelnut flour xxi, xxiii, 189, 192
hemp flour 189, 192
   milk xlii
Homemade Soft Pretzels 182
honey, sweeteners xxxix, xl
Honey Ginger Carrot Cakes with Lime Cream Cheese Frosting 64

Honey-Roasted Beet and
    Lemon Cheesecake 140
humidity, effect xlviii

I

ice cream, Teff-Crusted
    Ice Cream Over Grilled
    Peaches and Lavender
    Chamomile Syrup 149

K

kaniwa flour 189, 192
kasha, *see buckwheat*
kneading dough xxxv

L

lavender, Teff-Crusted Ice
    Cream Over Grilled
    Peaches and Lavender
    Chamomile Syrup 149
leavening agents xxxvii, xxxviii
lemon, Cranberry Lemon
    Millet Quinoa Squares 36
    Honey-Roasted Beet and
        Lemon Cheesecake 140
    Lemon Crepe Cake 86
    Lemon Quinoa Cream
        Pie 109
    Raspberry Lemon Quinoa
        and Oat Loaves 76
Light and Fluffy Cream
    Puffs 52
lime, Honey Ginger Carrot
    Cakes with Lime Cream
    Cheese Frosting 64
    Mashed Blueberry Lime
        Hand Pies 112
    Tangy Lime Greek Yogurt
        Pie 124
loaves 43
    Banana Breakfast Bread 70

Basil Pesto and Pine Nut
    Loaf 173
Breakfast Popover Loaf 71
Chocolate Swirl Banana
    Loaf 73
Prune Spice Loaf 72
Raspberry Lemon Quinoa
    and Oat Loaves 76
Roasted Red Pepper
    Loaf 175

M

Maple Raisin Cinnamon Buns
    74
maple syrup, sweeteners xxxix,
    xl
Mashed Blueberry Lime Hand
    Pies 112
marshmallow, Chocolate
    Whoopie Pies 21
    Espresso Cookie Bars with
        Honey Marshmallow
        Meringue 38
matcha, Mint Matcha
    Morsels 22
measuring xxx, xlviii
mesquite flour 189, 193
Milk Chocolate and Orange
    Blondies 39
millet *flour* xxvii, xxxiii
millet *flakes, flour, puffs, seeds* xxi,
    xxiii, xxxii, 189, 193
Mini Maple Cherry
    Cheesecakes 79
Mint Cherry Country Baked
    Biscuits 51
Mint Chocolate-Dipped
    Cake Bites 77
Mint Matcha Morsels 22
Mocha Crinkle Cookies 12
molasses, Ginger Squash
    Molasses Cookies 15

Molasses Ancient Grain
    Loaf 170
Monster Oat Chia Cookies 8
Montina flour 189, 193
mucilaginous properties xxv,
    xxxv, xxxvi
muffins 43
    Cranberry, Walnut and
        Rosemary Muffins 58
    Nut and Chocolate
        Muffins 62
    Strawberry Jam Oat
        Muffins 59
    Sweet Potato Muffins 60
    Wild Blueberry Buttermilk
        Bran Muffins 61
Multigrain Buns 178
muscovado, sweeteners
    xxxix, xl
myths, gluten-free baking xlviii

N

Nut and Chocolate Muffins 62
nut butter, Chocolate
    Hazelnut Brownies 41
    Milk Chocolate and Orange
        Blondies 39
    Praline Cheesecake
        Blondies 40
    White Chocolate, Orange
        and Nut Butter Quinoa
        Squares 32
nut flours xxi
nutrition xxi
nuts, Pressed Nut Crust 105

O

oatcakes, Cranberry Lemon
Oatcakes 50
Thyme, Rosemary and
Parmesan Oatcakes 49
oat *groats*, *flakes* xxi, xxiv
flour xxi, xxiv, xxviii, xxxiii,
189, 193
rolled xxxii
oats, Apple Raisin Oat
Squares 30
Chewy Raisin Oatmeal
Chia Cookies 6
Citrus Sorghum and
Oat Biscotti 24
Hawaiian Oat Squares 31
Oat Fig Newtons 18
Oat, Strawberry and Cream
Cheese Thumbprint
Cookies 7
Raspberry Lemon Quinoa
and Oat Loaves 76
oils, use in baking xlii
Old-Fashioned Cake-
Doughnuts 67
olive oil xlii

P

palm oil, organic xlii
papaya, Hawaiian Oat
Squares 31
Parmesan Salt and Pepper
Biscuits 55
pastry xlvi
Gluten-Free Pie
Pastry I 102
Gluten-Free Pie
Pastry II 103
Cream Cheese Pastry 104
pea flour (protein) xxi,
190, 193

peaches, Teff Crusted Ice
Cream Over Grilled
Peaches and Lavender
Chamomile Syrup 149
peanut flour 190, 193
peanut butter, Graham Peanut
Butter Chocolate Bites 156
Peanut Butter Chocolate
Chunk Cookies 11
Pecan Date Pie 120
pies 99
pineapple, Hawaiian Oat
Squares 31
Pineapple Citrus Berry Crisp
96
pine nut, Apricot, Walnut and
Pine Nut Granola Bars 29
Basil Pesto and Pine Nut
Loaf 173
potato flour xxi, 190, 193
potato starch xxi, xxiv,
190, 193
binder xxxv
pound cake, Ancient Grain 80
Praline Cheesecake
Blondies 40
Pressed Nut Crust 105
pretzels, Homemade Soft 182
prune, Chocolate, Walnut
and Prune Millet Quinoa
Squares 35
Prune Spice Loaf 72
psyllium husks xxxii, xliii,
190, 193
binder xxxiv, xxxv, xxxvi,
xlvi
pudding, Raisin Farmhouse 95
Sticky Toffee Pudding 144
Strawberry and Raspberry
Coconut Cream
Trifle 146
Yorkshire Pudding with
Roasted Strawberries
and Basil 133
puffs, Apricot, Walnut and
Pine Nut Granola Bars 32

Candied Ginger, Orange
and Pistachio Bark 153
Chocolate, Walnut and
Prune Millet Quinoa
Squares 35
Cranberry Lemon Millet
Quinoa Squares 36
Thai Coconut Dark
Chocolate Bark with
Lime Zest 152
White Chocolate, Orange
and Nut Butter Quinoa
Squares 32

Q

quinoa, Chocolate Quinoa
Pie 122
Fluffy White Quinoa
Cake 82
Lemon Quinoa Cream
Pie 109
Outrageous Quinoa
Chocolate Cake 91
Raspberry Lemon Quinoa
and Oat Loaves
quinoa *flakes, flour, puffs, seeds* xxi,
xxiv, xxxii, xxxiii, 190, 193

R

Raisin Farmhouse Pudding 95
raspberry, Rich Chocolate
Raspberry Tartlets 126
Strawberry and Raspberry
Coconut Cream
Trifle 146
Raspberry Lemon Quinoa
and Oat Loaves 76
red pepper, Roasted Red
Pepper Loaf 175
rice milk xlii
rice starch 190, 193
Rich Chocolate Raspberry
Tartlets 126

rising, yeast breads xlvi
Roasted Red Pepper Loaf 175

S

Salted Caramel Pecan
Shortbread Bites 17
scones, Toffee Maple Bacon 56
seaweed powder, binder xxxv
shortbread, Salted Caramel
Pecan Shortbread Bites 17
sorghum, *flour, grains* xxi, xxv,
xxxii, 190, 193
soybean (soy) flour xxi,
190, 193
soy milk xlii
squares 1
squash, Ginger Squash
Molasses Cookies 15
stabilizers, *see Binders and
Stabilizers*
starches, gluten-free xxi
Sticky Toffee Pudding 144
storage xxi, xlviii
strawberries, Oat, Strawberry
and Cream Cheese
Thumbprint Cookies 7
Strawberry and Raspberry
Coconut Cream
Trifle 146
Strawberry Jam Oat
Muffins 59
Strawberry Shortcakes with
Sweet Chantilly Cream 151
substitute, egg or fat xxxvi
Sucanat xxxix, xli
Sweet Potato Flour 190
Sweet Potato Muffins 60
sweet rice flour xxi, xxv,
191, 193
sweeteners xxxix

T

Tangy Lime Greek Yogurt
Pie 124
tapioca starch (flour) xxi, xxv,
191, 193
binder xxxv
tarts 99
Teff-Crusted Ice Cream
Over Grilled Peaches and
Lavender Chamomile
Syrup 149
teff *flour, grains* xxi, xxv, xxxiii,
191, 193
binder xxxv
Tender Egg Bread 166
Thai Coconut Dark Chocolate
Bark with Lime Zest 152
thermometer, oven and
instant read xliii
Thyme, Rosemary and
Parmesan Oatcakes 49
tips, gluten-free baking xlvi
toffee, Sticky Toffee
Pudding 144
Toffee Maple Bacon Scones 56
tofu, binder xxxv
tortilla, Ancient Grain
Tortilla Wraps 176
Triple Chocolate Coconut
Chia Cookies 16
truffles, Cherry Almond 154
turbinado sugar xxxix, xli

V

vegan alternatives, binders xxxv

W

wafers, Graham-Style 46
walnuts, Apricot, Walnut and
Pine Nut Granola Bars 29
Cranberry, Walnut and
Rosemary Muffins 58

weighing flours xxx
Wild Blueberry Buttermilk
Bran Muffins 61
White Chocolate, Orange
and Nut Butter Quinoa
Squares 32
White Dinner Buns 180
white rice flour xxi, xxv,
191, 193
wild rice flour 191
wraps, Ancient Grain
Tortilla 176

X

xanthan gum xxxiv, xxxv, xxxvi,
xlvi, 191, 193

Y

yeast xxxvii
yeast breads xlvi
yogurt, Tangy Lime Greek
Yogurt Pie 124
Yogurt Cut-Out
Cookies 134
Yorkshire Pudding with
Roasted Strawberries
and Basil 133

Z

zucchini, Double-Layer
Chocolate Chia Zucchini
Cake 138

Happy Baking!

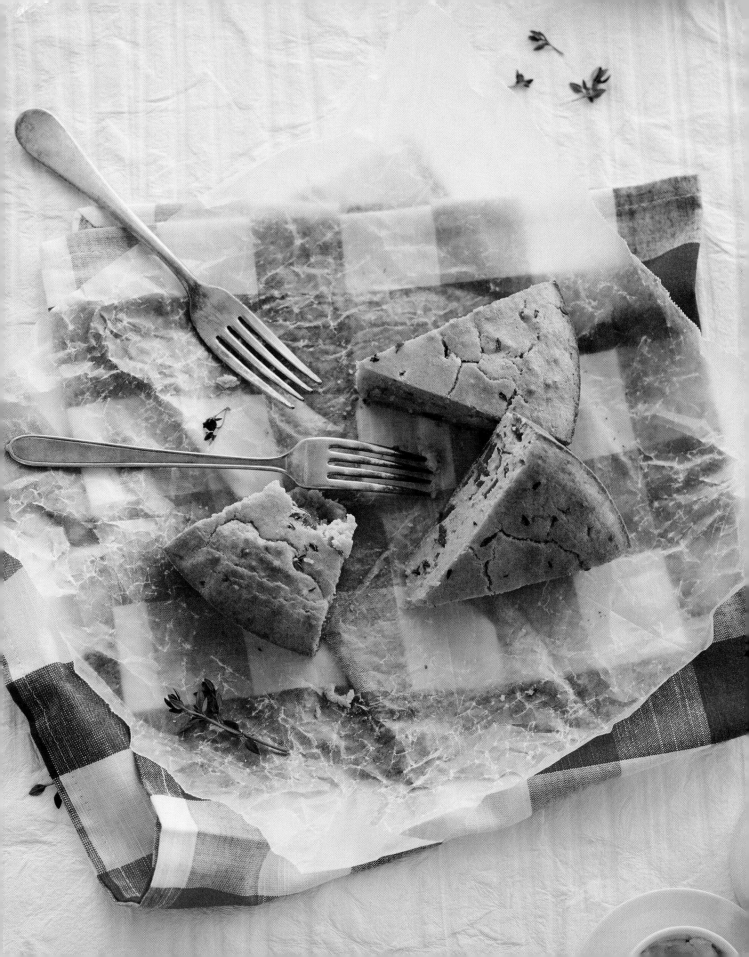

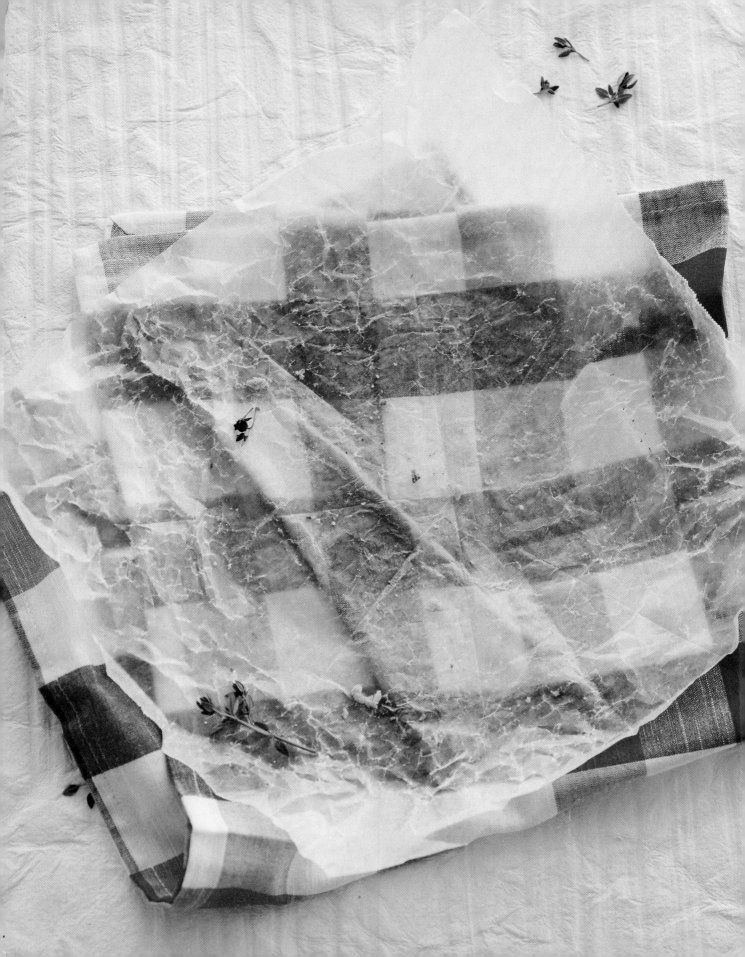